RAISING S
INTELLIGI

Many parents feel uncomfortable with the thought of having 'the talk' with their children, especially teenagers. But what many people don't realise is how much of sexuality education has nothing to do with sex itself.

In this book, Clinical Sexologist Anisa Varasteh teaches the foundations of a comprehensive sexuality education for children and teenagers and answers the most common questions young people have about sex and sexuality. Contrary to popular belief, talking about sex and sexuality does not make young people more prone to sexual experimentation. This book provides research-based evidence for how a comprehensive sexuality education is important for children's safety and psychological and physical well-being. It identifies the barriers to having open conversations with children and teenagers, and outlines methods for how to overcome them. With a focus on skills, the book addresses the building blocks of sexuality education and how to develop an environment of mutual trust; it outlines key topics for discussion and the skills that children need to develop to make healthy decisions about their sexuality.

Complete with practical support, including over 20 worksheets and a comprehensive list of tough questions from teenagers—and suggestions for how to address them—this book is an essential resource for parents, carers and educators who are responsible for the health, safety and development of children and teenagers.

Anisa Varasteh is a Clinical Sexologist, the Director of Relate Sexology and the President of the Society of Australian Sexologists (SA/NT branch). Anisa provides therapy to individuals and partners as well as consultancy and training on mental health- and sexuality-related topics to clinicians and organisations.

RAISING SEXUALLY INTELLIGENT KIDS

PRACTICAL SKILLS FOR PARENTS, CARERS AND EDUCATORS

Anisa Varasteh

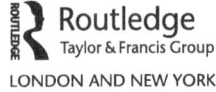

LONDON AND NEW YORK

Designed cover image: © Getty Images

First published 2024
by Routledge
4 Park Square, Milton Park, Abingdon, Oxon OX14 4RN

and by Routledge
605 Third Avenue, New York, NY 10158

Routledge is an imprint of the Taylor & Francis Group, an informa business

© 2024 Anisa Varasteh

The right of Anisa Varasteh to be identified as author of this work has been asserted in accordance with sections 77 and 78 of the Copyright, Designs and Patents Act 1988.

All rights reserved. No part of this book may be reprinted or reproduced or utilised in any form or by any electronic, mechanical, or other means, now known or hereafter invented, including photocopying and recording, or in any information storage or retrieval system, without permission in writing from the publishers.

Trademark notice: Product or corporate names may be trademarks or registered trademarks, and are used only for identification and explanation without intent to infringe.

British Library Cataloguing-in-Publication Data
A catalogue record for this book is available from the British Library

Library of Congress Cataloging-in-Publication Data
Names: Varasteh, Anisa, author.
Title: Raising sexually intelligent kids : practical skills for parents, carers and educators / Anisa Varasteh.
Description: Abingdon, Oxon ; New York, NY : Routledge, 2024. | Includes bibliographical references.
Identifiers: LCCN 2023025804 (print) | LCCN 2023025805 (ebook) | ISBN 9781032557489 (hardback) | ISBN 9781032564531 (paperback) | ISBN 9781003435600 (ebook)
Subjects: LCSH: Sex instruction for children. | Children and sex. | Children—Sexual behavior. | Parenting.
Classification: LCC HQ57 .V37 2024 (print) | LCC HQ57 (ebook) | DDC 372.37/2—dc23/eng/20230802
LC record available at https://lccn.loc.gov/2023025804
LC ebook record available at https://lccn.loc.gov/2023025805

ISBN: 978-1-032-55748-9 (hbk)
ISBN: 978-1-032-56453-1 (pbk)
ISBN: 978-1-003-43560-0 (ebk)

DOI: 10.4324/9781003435600

Typeset in Palatina and Scala Sans
by Apex CoVantage, LLC

For Luna, my littlest muse, who sprinkles fairy dust on my life and imagination.

Contents

List of worksheets	ix
Acknowledgements	x
Introduction	1

PART 1
Foundations of sexuality education   11

1	Why is talking about sexuality with children important?	13
2	Why is talking about sex with children awkward?	27
3	Foundations of sexuality education	48

PART 2
Sexual intelligence skills   55

4	Attachment styles and their role in adulthood relationships	57
5	Emotional intelligence skills	66
6	A strength-based approach	109
7	Value-based decision-making	113
8	Healthy boundaries	126

Contents

PART 3
Topics to talk about with children   **147**

9   What topics to talk about?   149

10   Provide a balanced and realistic view of sex   165

11   Include pleasure in your conversation about sexuality   168

12   Gender and sexual identity   171

13   Body image   186

14   Age-based tips for conversations   191

15   Identifying and responding to sexual abuse in children   199

Appendix 1- Navigating adolescence: answers to real-life questions from teenagers   213
Appendix 2- List of age-appropriate sexuality books for children and young people   238
Index   242

Worksheets

1.1	Definition of sexuality	23
1.2	Your motivation	25
2.1	What influenced your sexuality?	29
2.2	Internalised sexual beliefs	32
2.3	Attitude towards sex	34
2.4	Your relationship with pleasure	36
2.5	Identifying triggers	39
5.1	Identifying emotions	70
5.2	Exploring and identifying emotions	73
5.3	Anger management for children	84
5.4	Anger stop signs	85
5.5	What to do with my anger	86
7.1	Identifying times when you were authentic	116
7.2	Identifying your drives	117
7.3	Identifying who you admire	117
7.4	Determining your top values	118
7.5	Prioritising your top values	120
7.6	Revaluating your values	121
7.7	Value-based communication	124
8.1	Where do your boundaries come from?	130
8.2	Identifying your boundaries	133
8.3	Healthy messages for boundary building	136

Acknowledgements

I am incredibly grateful to the following individuals for their invaluable support in making this book a reality: Arteen Ramezani, Nicole Boughton, and Samantha Seymour, thank you for taking the time to read my book and providing me with insightful feedback that greatly improved the flow of the book.

Big thanks to Amanda Mountford, my dear friend and Communications Manager, for being my hype woman and using her hawk-like proofreading skills to make my work shine like a diamond.

A special shout-out to my brother, Samim, for dealing with the mind-numbing task of referencing. You spared me from the agony of doing what I dread the most about writing a book!

To my partner, Viktor. Your unwavering support and insights have been like fuel to my engine—I couldn't have done it without you! Your belief in me has kept me going when my motivation was as low as my caffeine levels. Thanks for being my cheerleader, sounding board, and all-around amazing partner.

I want to give a big shoutout to my partner-in-crime, Melody Grobitsch—my oldest and bestest friend. Thank you for always being there for me when I needed someone to talk to about my sexuality, even when you didn't quite understand it yourself. And thank you for reading my book and providing me with feedback that helped me perfect my prose.

I would also like to extend my appreciation to the groups of parents and teenagers who generously shared their

Acknowledgements

experiences and questions with me. Your input has enriched the content of my book and added valuable perspectives.

Last but certainly not least, a massive shout-out to my dad for being an absolute legend during the final months of publishing my book. Your assistance in taking care of our little bundle of joy, Luna, was a true lifesaver. Thanks for being there for Luna when I couldn't, and for making sure that she was safe and happy while I was busy typing away like a mad person. Your help and love for our daughter mean more to me than words can express. You're the best, Baba!

Introduction

When should I start talking to my child about sex?

How much detail should I provide when discussing sex with my child?

How would I know if a sexual behaviour is normal or not?

How can I teach my child about consent and healthy relationships?

What should I do if my child asks a question I'm not comfortable answering?

What should I do when I see them playing 'doctors'?

Should I talk to my child about pornography, and if so, how?

How can I address issues related to gender and sexuality with my child?

How can I minimise the risk of sexual abuse in my children?

What resources can I use to support my child's sex education?

These are the most common questions parents have about sexuality education for their children. By the end of this book you will have the answer to these questions and many more!

But firstly, congratulations on taking an important step towards your child's well-being and sense of fulfilment! You may have had a comprehensive sexuality education as a young person and would like to do the same for your child. You may not have had the opportunity to learn about sexuality in a positive and empowering way and you would like to gift this precious opportunity to your young person; or you may already have a lot of information and knowledge about sexuality and sex to share with your child, but not sure how to counteract the conflicting and harmful messages they receive from the environment on a daily basis. This book is for you.

We receive messages about sex and sexuality from the moment we are conceived. That's right, even before we are born. From 'gender reveal' parties, to choosing the colour of baby clothing, the toys, the name that is chosen for us, we are born into a pre-conceived idea of how our family and environment expects us to behave in relation to our sex, gender and sexuality. These messages are then reinforced by the interactions we have with the people in our lives. We learn from a very early age what body parts are 'private' or that touching certain parts of the body in front of others is not acceptable (or is even punishable), and we learn we cannot talk about certain things openly in public (or ever at all).

Based on my professional experience I believe humans, men, women and all other genders have a lot more similarities than differences. However, most of us are born in societies where there are two inflexible categories of gender, and we are treated differently based on the assumptions our parents and medical professionals make about our gender. Research shows girls are socialised to be modest, nice and 'pretty'. These traditional gender roles do not encourage women to be confident, assertive and speak their minds and communicate about their needs, especially in a sexual context.[1] Boys are limited in other ways by societal expectations of masculinity. 'Boys don't cry' or 'Boys are always strong' teach our young boys that vulnerability and expression of emotions are weaknesses. Yet, vulnerability and the ability to feel and express the full range of human emotions are two fundamental elements of a healthy and loving relationship. The unfortunate cost of such expectations and gender roles, for all genders, are high rates of depression, anxiety, domestic violence and suicide (Granato et al., 2015; King et al., 2020; Nowotny et al., 2015).

Young children are exposed to stories about bodies, marriage, love, privacy, birth, menstruation, sexual feelings, shame, being a boy or a girl and friendship from the media, games, fairy tales, family and friends. These messages influence their capacity to manage their sense of identity and relationships as they grow. But this is all inevitable. As humans living in a society, we cannot fully isolate ourselves from the environment we live in. We are influenced by it, we are shaped by it. But the good news is as parents and caregivers our influence on our children is much more significant than those of others in their life.

Your child is receiving information about sex and sexuality from their environment on a daily basis. As the saying goes: "if you are not talking to your children about sexuality someone else is."

In Australia the average age of children being exposed to pornography for the first time is eight years old (Parliament of Australia, 2021)! Just under half (44%) of Australian children aged 9–16 surveyed had encountered sexual images in the last month (Australian Government—Australian Institute of Family Studies, 2021). It's not a matter of if a child will see pornography but when.

Given that pornography's design and intention is not sex education and therefore is not an accurate representation of safe, consensual and pleasurable sex, it is unfortunate that in the absence of quality and effective sexuality education many children seek pornography to learn about sex, sexuality, fantasies and relationships. I am not anti-porn. I believe watching pornography when not used for education can be entertaining, fun and exciting, just like Hollywood movies (more on this later).

Introduction

> **Some statistics about sexuality education, teens and their parents (Center for Family Life Education, 2003)**
>
> - Teenagers who have talked with their parents about sexual matters become sexually active later than those who haven't.
> - Most parents (90%) rate themselves as approachable on the topic of sexuality but only 74% of teenagers agree.
> - One in five parents think that their teen is sexually active but in reality about one-third of teenagers claim to be. At the same time, 13% of parents admit they wouldn't know whether their teen was sexually active or not.
> - In general more parents think they have had 'the talk' about sexual health than teens do (80% vs 73%), with 20% of parents admitting that they have never had the conversation with their teen.

As parents, we play a crucial role in shaping our children's understanding of healthy relationships. Children learn by observing, and their primary source of learning is from the behaviour they witness from their parents or caregivers. Therefore, it is essential for parents to model positive relationships to their children.

Children observe and learn from their parents' interactions and relationships. If parents demonstrate positive behaviour towards each other, their children will also learn how to interact with others in a positive manner. On the other hand, if parents model unhealthy relationships, children may also adopt negative behaviour and attitudes towards relationships.

That's why a significant part of this book focuses on how you as parents or caregivers can improve your relational and emotional skills. By honing these skills, you can model positive relationships, which in turn will help your child develop the skills they need to build healthy and positive relationships themselves. Children who grow up in homes where positive relationships are modelled tend to have more fulfilling relationships as adults. They are more likely to develop empathy, communication skills and problem-solving abilities that are critical for maintaining healthy relationships.

Providing a secure and stable home environment is crucial in providing sexuality education to children. This allows parents to provide accurate and age-appropriate information, which helps children make informed decisions about their sexual health. When children feel comfortable talking to their parents about sex, they are less likely to seek information from unreliable sources such as peers or the internet, reducing the risk of experimentation or misinformation.

It's important to note that modelling positive relationships isn't just about showing affection towards your partner or spouse. It also includes demonstrating healthy conflict resolution, respectful communication, empathy towards others and other relationship skills. By modelling these behaviours, parents can help their children develop the tools they need to navigate difficult situations and build strong relationships.

Sounds like a big task? This is why I have written this book, to support you through this wonderful, confusing, heartbreaking, joyful and mysterious journey of parenting. Together with the latest psychology research and information, your wisdom, life experience, intuition and resilience we can teach your child/children the skills they need to make safe and enjoyable decisions about their sexuality and relationships.

In each section I have attempted to provide you with examples of how a particular skill could relate to healthy sexual and/or romantic relationships or used when having conversations about sexuality with young people.

In the first section of the book I will discuss the foundation of sexuality education, because as you will see in Part 2 the skills we teach our kids to make decisions and interact with others is much more important than the facts and figures we share with them. In the second part I will talk

Introduction

about the topics you need to cover when providing a comprehensive sexuality education for your child. Throughout the book you will see a collection of real-life questions by parents and my responses to them. The list of questions and parenting scenarios are endless, so I invite you to use these as a guide to talk with your child. I hope you customise them to fit the unique needs of your child and family as a complement to the existing tools and knowledge you already have. In using the example answers I have given it is important not to worry so much about the exact words I have used but to embody validation and curiosity when responding to your child's questions.

For now, once again, congratulations on taking this important step towards your child's well-being and fulfilment. If you get confused, overwhelmed or anxious at times, don't forget that you are not alone. Do what you need to take care of yourself, talk with a trusted friend/partner, do something enjoyable for self-care and know that you are on the right path.

If you are ready, let's begin!

SOME THINGS TO CONSIDER WHILE READING THIS BOOK

Language
I have written this book with the aim of providing the tools parents and caregivers and educators need regardless of their gender identity and sexual orientation. I have intended to be as inclusive of all gender identities, sexualities and relationship structures as possible. I use gender-neutral pronouns to refer to children and young people (they, their, theirs) as well as gender-neutral language when describing body parts, as genitals don't define our gender (more on this later), and sometimes I use the term 'people with a penis/vulva'. Unless specified, when I use the terms 'man' and 'woman', 'boy' or 'girl' I am including everyone who identifies with these terms—not just cisgendered people.

I use the word 'partner' to refer to whoever the person is having sex with. I prefer the word partner (instead of husband, wife, boyfriend, girlfriend, sweetheart, lover, etc.) because not only does it apply to all genders, but because it could mean someone you just met or the person you have been in a relationship with for 25 years.

Universality
The frameworks I have provided in this book have been applied by people across countries and cultures, and they have a level of universality. However, I would like to acknowledge that most of the frameworks used in this book are based on research done in Western countries and are not the only way we can view human psychology and sexuality.

Diversity of experiences
I have attempted to provide a broad spectrum of voices and experiences in this book. I have conducted interviews, focus groups and surveys with parents and caregivers spanning a range of sexualities, genders, ages, cultures and life experiences. Also the questions asked by teens are based on surveys I conducted with youth and young adults about questions they wish they knew the answers to when they were teenagers.

Confidentiality
I have used client experiences and stories throughout the book to give you examples of what the techniques and strategies can look like in real life. I have removed any identifiable details and have changed client names to ensure their privacy.

Self-care
Sex can be a challenging topic for various reasons. Maybe being sexually vulnerable in the past has led to emotional pain; perhaps some aspects of your body make you feel vulnerable; maybe your past or current relationship were sources of self-doubt or stress or maybe you have experienced

trauma which complicates your relationships with sexuality. Please honour your needs and attend to them as you read this book. My aim is to leave you feeling more confident to raise sexually intelligent children. And I really hope you have fun reading this book!

Structure

As you dive into the chapters of the book, you may notice a variation in their lengths, with some being more extensive than others. We wanted to give special attention to the foundation-building and crucial skills children need to make informed choices about their sexual and relational lives. That's why these chapters take a little more time to explore and discuss. On the other hand, we have condensed topics like considerations for providing sexuality education to children, making them easily digestible while still delivering important insights. Our goal is to provide you with a practical and comprehensive guide that covers all aspects of raising sexually intelligent kids, ensuring their well-being and fostering positive attitudes towards sexuality. Together, let's embark on this exciting and important journey!

REFERENCE LIST

Australian Government—Australian Institute of Family Studies. (2021). The effects of pornography on children and young people. *Australian Institute of Family Studies*. Retrieved May 12, 2021, from https://aifs.gov.au/publications/effects-pornography-children-and-young-people-snapshot

Center for Family Life Education. (2003). *Talk soon. Talk often. A guide for parents talking to their kids about sex.*

Granato, S. L., Smith, P. N., & Selwyn, C. N. (2015). Acquired capability and masculine gender norm adherence: Potential pathways to higher rates of male suicide. *Psychology of Men & Masculinity, 16*(3), 246–253. https://doi.org/10.1037/a0038181

Herman, J., Haas, A., & Rodgers, P. (2014). *Suicide attempts among transgender and gender non-conforming adults.* American Foundation for Suicide Prevention.

King, T., Shields, M., Sojo, V., Daraganova, G., Currier, D., O'Neil, A., King, K., & Milner, A. (2020). Expressions of masculinity and associations with suicidal ideation among young males. *BMC Psychiatry*, *20*(1), 228–228. https://doi.org/10.1186/s12888-020-2475-y

Nowotny, K. M., Peterson, R. L., & Boardman, J. D. (2015). Gendered contexts: Variation in suicidal ideation by female and male youth across U.S. states. *Journal of Health and Social Behavior*, *56*(1), 114–130. https://doi.org/10.1177/0022146514568350

Parliament of Australia. (2021). 3. Age verification for online pornography—Parliament of Australia. *Aph.gov.au*. Retrieved May 12, 2021, from www.aph.gov.au/Parliamentary_Business/Committees/House/Social_Policy_and_Legal_Affairs/Online-ageverification/Report/section?id=committees%2Freportrep%2F024436%2F72615

Part 1
Foundations of sexuality education

CHAPTER 1

Why is talking about sexuality with children important?

Talking about sexuality with children improves their physical and mental well-being and reduces the risk of sexual assault.

A research conducted in 2017 shows 68% of the participants (teenagers) engaged in vaginal sex and oral sex and 22% in vaginal, oral and anal sex. Only 34% of these teenagers used condoms in their last vaginal intercourse and 47% in their last anal intercourse (Chow et al., 2017).

This means 66% of them did not use a condom for vaginal intercourse and 47% didn't use a condom for anal intercourse. Most parents find these numbers concerning. Anal sex in particular has a higher transmission of STIs (sexually transmitted infections), including HIV, primarily because the anus has more fragile tissue and does not self-lubricate. Small tears are much more likely to occur and therefore expose the blood to risk of infection. But how can talking about sex help?

Contrary to public belief, talking about sex and sexuality does not make young people more prone to sexual experimentation. It is in fact an important factor in keeping children safe from sexual, physical and psychological harm (United Nations Population Fund, 2021). Not talking about sexuality and a lack of comprehensive sex education makes young people vulnerable to coercion, unintended pregnancy and STIs (United Nations Population Fund, 2021).

Based on the latest scientific evidence (United Nations Population Fund, 2021; Family Planning Victoria, 2016), sexuality education:

- Helps young people become more responsible in their attitude and behaviour regarding sexual and reproductive health.
- Is crucial in addressing the issue of girls dropping out of school due to teenage pregnancy and related reproductive health concerns.
- Does not lead to increased sexual activity, risky sexual behaviours or rates of STI/HIV infections.
- Shows that abstinence-only programmes are ineffective in preventing early sexual initiation or reducing the frequency of sexual activity and number of partners among young people.
- Delays the onset of first sexual experience.

Comprehensive sex education has been found to have numerous benefits beyond preventing teenage pregnancy and STIs. One of the most significant benefits is its potential to prevent child sexual abuse. By teaching young people about healthy boundaries, consent and the signs of abusive behaviour, comprehensive sex education can empower young people to recognise and report abuse (Goldfarb & Lieberman, 2021).

Additionally, comprehensive sex education can create a sense of safety and improve mental health outcomes for LGBTQI+ young people. By including information on sexual orientation, gender identity and LGBTQI+ issues, sex education can help LGBTQI+ youth feel seen, valued and supported. This can lead to improved mental health outcomes, including decreased rates of depression, anxiety and suicidal ideation (Goldfarb & Lieberman, 2021).

Finally, comprehensive sex education has been found to reduce rates of relationship violence. By teaching young people about healthy relationships, communication skills and the importance of consent, sexuality education can help prevent the development of abusive behaviours and promote healthy relationships. This can lead to decreased rates of domestic violence, intimate partner violence and sexual assault (Goldfarb & Lieberman, 2021).

Chris Harley, president and CEO of SIECUS, emphasises the positive impacts of sex education:

> At SIECUS: Sex Ed for Social Change, we have been asserting that individual and social benefits of sex education extend far beyond simply decreasing rates of unintended pregnancies and sexually transmitted infections among young people. This new wealth of research is just the start of illuminating that the power and importance of comprehensive, inclusive sex education is in its ability to do so much more. The findings are clear: **sex education helps all of our young people lead happier, healthier, safer lives—no matter who they are or how they identify**.
> (Advocates for Youth, 2020)

As a clinical sexologist, I have personally witnessed the significance of comprehensive sexuality education in correcting misconceptions and myths about sexuality. Throughout my professional and personal life, I have encountered many young people and adults who hold inaccurate beliefs about sexual health and behaviour. Some of the common myths and misconceptions about sexuality are:

- Masturbation is only for boys/men, periods are for girls/women.
- Periods are gross.
- If you are a girl, you need to understand there is a fine line between being a slut and being a prude and your job is to stay right in the middle.
- Sexual pleasure is mainly for men. If the woman has pain, she will have to tolerate it and find a way to deal with it.
- Sex is penetration of a penis in a vagina.
- 'Losing your virginity' will be painful, and there is nothing you can do about it.
- Men have high sexual drive and women intrinsically have lower libido.
- Young girls are more vulnerable to sexual assault than young boys.

- Only men can have 'sexual dysfunctions'.
- Sex has an important meaning attached to it. Having it or not having it says something about who you are as a person.
- My partner should just know what I want/like.
- My partner wants what I am doing.
- Asking for consent kills the mood.
- You haven't had 'real sex' until a penis has gone into a vagina.

We will examine some of these myths in more detail later, but you can see how these ideas can lead to confusion, dissatisfaction, disappointment and unfortunately emotional hurt and even sexual assault.

YOUNG PEOPLE WANT TO TALK ABOUT SEXUALITY WITH THEIR PARENTS

Research shows that young people want to talk with their parents/carers about relationships and sexuality, but many parents/caregivers may feel uncomfortable about having these conversations. By being honest and open, your young person is more likely to turn to you for accurate information and answers to their questions. This reduces their risk of being in an unhealthy relationship, of experiencing unwanted sex or an unintended pregnancy or of getting a sexually transmissible infection (STI) (Family Planning Victoria, 2016).

It is interesting for most people to know that children and young people who are raised in homes where they can talk about sexuality openly with at least with one adult are at a lower risk of sexual assault. Why? Let me tell you the story of one of my clients. Let's call her Kate. Kate was in a relationship with a loving partner for three years. She came to see me because she could not feel any sexual pleasure, although she loved her partner dearly and they had a healthy and functioning relationship. After a few sessions, Kate disclosed to me about a history of childhood sexual assault that she had been subjected to at the age of eight. The perpetrator was her horse-riding instructor. Without going into disturbing details, the assault had gone on over eight months. Kate said as much as her parents were loving and caring, they never talked about sex and sexuality openly at home. It was a topic that she had learnt was not to be talked about. It was shameful and embarrassing.

> Sex was never mentioned at home. I knew it was shameful to touch my genitals or talk about anything related to 'It'. It didn't even cross my mind to tell my parents because it was way out of line. We never talked about 'It'. I just remember feeling this massive shame, this feeling that I had done something wrong to bring my family shame.

We all know that eight-year-old Kate had done nothing wrong. She was unfortunately in the proximity of a rapist and a child molester. However, it could have been stopped much earlier if Kate were able to understand and communicate with her parents what was going on. When Kate's parents found out about the assault 12 years later, they were shattered. They could not bear the thought that unknowingly they had put their child at an increased risk of sexual assault and trauma.

Unfortunately, Kate's story is not a unique story. As a mental health practitioner and sexologist, I have heard too many similar stories of young people of *all genders* not being able to communicate with their parents about sexual assault, unintended pregnancy or being stuck in an unhealthy relationship.

By talking about sexuality openly and comfortably we foster an environment for our children to approach us about anything they may find confusing, confronting or uncomfortable. By creating a relationship based on mutual trust we increase the possibility of being the first point of call for our children when they feel scared or vulnerable. No one wants to find out second-hand what trauma their child has experienced or to find out when it is too late.

According to the Department of Education and Early Childhood Development (2021), important messages and skills that contribute to children's safety include:

- Teaching children about the proper names of their body parts.
- Giving children permission to talk and ask questions about sexual body parts.
- Explaining the qualities of respectful relationships.
- Identifying a support network of teachers and adults to whom they could turn (in case you are unavailable).
- Understanding personal safety, that is, safety for their bodies and how to keep themselves safe.

CHILDREN ARE ALREADY RECEIVING MESSAGES ABOUT SEXUALITY, GENDER AND RELATIONSHIPS FROM THEIR ENVIRONMENT

Home and family environment

Home is the first place for a child to learn about feeling safe, close and connected. The family environment provides opportunities for lots of moments to teach children about bodies, sexuality, gender roles and relationships. Teaching children about sexuality starts with everyday activities such as bathing, understanding appropriate times for nudity and learning about body parts. Allowing children to ask questions about their bodies, relationships and gender is an important aspect of sexuality education. As children get older questions about sex and the experiences of first love and romantic relationships offer additional opportunities for learning about sexuality. Children also learn by observing their parents' and caregivers' reactions to others' relationships, gender expressions and expectations of gender roles. Seemingly benign jokes and conversations about sexual assault or an acquaintance's sexual orientation or relationship structure teaches our children about the values we hold around sexuality and can contribute to them feeling safe or unsafe to come to us when they have questions or when they feel upset or threatened by something.

School

Apart from stories that are shared on the playground, children learn about sexuality in the way the schools manage everyday situations, for example, a teacher's reaction when someone gets their period at school or if two young children are found showing each other their genitals, how teachers address and respond to questions and discussions about sexuality in the classroom, even simple things like school uniform expectations of gender expressions at school.

Changing rooms and playgrounds can be a place that foster a sense of belonging, satisfying children's typical curiosity, or they can be a place of bullying and body-shaming. These all contribute to the way children view sexuality and feel about their own bodies and sexuality.

During high school, many students begin to have their first romantic and sexual relationships. The formal sexuality education provided by schools can have a significant impact on a young person's confidence to make informed decisions about their bodies and sexuality.

Finding out what children learn at school about sexuality (formally and informally) can be a great conversation starter at home.

Media

Pause for a moment and consider the amount of media that you encounter in a single day, whether it be watching TV and movies; browsing the internet; reading newspapers, books and magazines; listening to music and music videos or playing video games. Considering the amount of advertisements encountered during media consumption, it's not surprising that media has a strong impact on our perspectives, attitudes, values and world view, particularly regarding sexuality. Media messages play a key role in shaping how kids feel about their bodies, gender norms and ideas about sex.

A simple example of how our sexuality is constructed and shaped by the media is Disney movies. Reflect on the Disney movies you watched when you were a child. These movies usually centre around a young, dominant male character such as a prince, a colonial ship captain or a soldier who becomes romantically interested in a young woman. It is always assumed that both characters are heterosexual and, in the end, the woman falls in love with the man and they get married. Children can learn a lot about gender and sexuality from these movies, particularly about the importance of traditional ideas of masculine and feminine behaviour (Kang et al., 2019).

Apart from the overt messages movies send about relationships, romance, sexuality, gender and so on, there are many subtle ways we learn about these concepts. I would like you to take a moment and think about the overt and covert messages your child receives about sexuality from their environment. Remember sexuality is anything related to gender, gender expression, love, romance, consent, respect, pleasure and so on.

The question is not whether children will learn about sex and sexuality but what and where they learn from.

Here are some other examples:

- Men love sports and women love getting their nails done (but women don't like sports and men don't like getting their nails done).
- Women are sensitive, dependent, fragile, dutiful, resigned and timid.
- Boys like trucks and girls like dolls (but boys don't like dolls and girls don't like trucks).
- Everyone needs an opposite-sex partner to spend their life with.

Table 1.1 displays the most common messages children/young people receive from their environment (mainstream media, peers, broader society, etc.) and the impact on their sexuality as adults. Do any of them resonate with you and your experience?

Why is talking about sexuality with children important?

Table 1.1 Common messages received by children from their surroundings

Overt message	Covert message	Impact
Boys don't cry.	Showing emotions is a sign of weakness and lack of masculinity.	Boys/men not being able to express emotions is unhealthy and is a factor in mental illness later in life. It has also been known as a factor in suicide due to the shame associated with seeking help and feeling 'weak'.
Girls are pretty. Boys are strong.	Girls/women are valued for their physical appearance and boys/men for their strength and internal characteristics.	Girls/women becoming overly engaged with physical appearance and not pursuing interests/passions which are focused on internal strength/characteristics. Men/boys feeling pressured to present as 'strong' all the time and this burden leading to toxic masculinity and mental health issues.
Women cook at home. Men pay for dinner when going out.	Domestic chores are intrinsically a woman's job. Men need to be the 'breadwinner' and main provider of the family.	Girls and women not exploring their potentials outside of 'house chores'. Men feeling pressured to financially provide for their partner and family. These gender roles and expectations can hinder people making decisions which are value-based and authentic.
Most/all relationships are between a man and a woman.	A lack of healthy representation of non-heterosexual relationships in the media can lead to children/people viewing non-heterosexuality as abnormal, wrong or least not as 'normal' as heterosexual relationships.	This view of sexual orientation can lead to homophobia in heterosexual children/people and internalised homophobia and mental health issues in non-heterosexual children/people.

(Continued)

Foundations of sexuality education

Table 1.1 Continued

Overt message	Covert message	Impact
Men always initiating sex or explicitly expressing sexual desire. Women presenting as reserved and only responding to a man's desire.	Men always need to be ready for sex and want sex regardless of the context and circumstances. Women intrinsically have lower libido than men and need to wait for a man to initiate a sexual behaviour. Women who initiate sex or express their desire overtly are sluts. There is something wrong with men who are not interested in sex ALL the time.	The pressure of being hypersexual can lead to men developing a variety of sexual dysfunctions, including erectile dysfunction, premature ejaculation or orgasm issues. Women can feel inhibited to express what is pleasurable for them out of the fear of 'slut shaming'. This can lead to pain and desire disorders in many women.

What is sexuality?

Most often when we hear the word 'sexuality' we think about sex—the physiological act of having sex. However, sexuality is much broader than sex. Sexuality is anything related to romantic and sexual relationships, puberty, changing bodies, respect, pleasure, body image, thoughts and beliefs, values, communication skills, sexual orientation, gender identity, gender and sexual expression, empathy, feeling safe in relation to your sexuality and much more.

For many people this way of looking at sexuality is a paradigm shift. When we understand sexuality is a broad spectrum of topics, we realise that our children are already receiving sexuality education ALL THE TIME: from us as well as from their environment. Even if you haven't talked to your child or young person about 'sex' yet, you have already provided them with some sexuality information. This book invites you to continue to do so with more awareness and intentionality. There are multiple opportunities throughout the day and week for us to talk about 'being a boy' or 'respecting other's boundaries' or 'families' with our children or share our values around respectful relationships. This is all sexuality education!

Worksheet 1.1   Definition of sexuality

Write down what other topics would fall under this broad definition of sexuality.

What is your motivation?

I would like to invite you to think about the following question: What is my motivation for reading this book? Take a few minutes to reflect and take notes. This can function as your compass in the future. It will be helpful in the times when you feel demotivated, confused or frustrated by either the environment, your young person's reactions, your own behaviour or others' comments.

Once you identify your True North (your motivation) you can reflect on the following to identify what the next step may be for you.

Worksheet 1.2 Your motivation

- How would you like things to be different?

- How would you **feel** if you knew your child had the skills to make safe and informed decisions about their life?

- On a scale of 1–10, how **ready** do you feel to have conversations with your child about sexuality?

- What led you to choose this specific number on the scale versus a lower number? (For example, if you chose 4 why didn't you choose 3? Write down your reason).

- On a scale of 1–10, how **confident** do you feel to have conversations with your child about sexuality?

- What led you to choose this specific number on the scale versus a lower number? (For example, if you chose 4 why didn't you choose 3? Write down your reason).

- What would you need to go one level higher?

- Who could offer you support in this journey?

REFERENCE LIST

Advocates for Youth. (2020). New research: Quality sex education has broad, long-term benefits for young people's' physical and mental health—advocates for youth. *Advocates for Youth*. Retrieved May 12, 2021, from https://www.advocatesforyouth.org/press-releases/new-research-quality-sex-education-has-broad-long-term-benefits-for-young-peoples-physical-and-mental-health/

Chow, E., Wigan, R., McNulty, A., Bell, C., Johnson, M., Marshall, L., Regan, D., Owen, L., Brotherton, J., Bradshaw, C., Fairley, C., Russell, D., & Chen, M. (2017). Early sexual experiences of teenage heterosexual males in Australia: A cross-sectional survey. *BMJ Open*, 7(10), e016779. https://doi.org/10.1136/bmjopen-2017-016779

Family Planning Victoria. (2016). Sex education for schools Melbourne | sex Ed in Melbourne | sex education services Melbourne | teaching sex in schools Melbourne. *Family Planning Victoria*. Retrieved May 12, 2021, from https://www.fpv.org.au/for-you/education/sex-education-talking-to-young-people

Goldfarb, E., & Lieberman, L. (2021). Three decades of research: The case for comprehensive sex education. *Journal of Adolescent Health*, 68(1), 13–27. https://doi.org/10.1016/j.jadohealth.2020.07.036

Kang, S., Lessard, D., & Heston, M. (2019). Media. In M. Heston, D. Lessard, & S. Kang (Eds.), *Introduction to women, gender, sexuality studies* (pp. 62–78). Libretexts.

United Nations Population Fund. (2021). Comprehensive sexuality education. *Unfpa.org*. Retrieved May 12, 2021, from https://www.unfpa.org/comprehensive-sexuality-education

Victoria State Government. (2021). Catching on early: Sexuality education for Victorian primary schools—FUSE—Department of Education & Training. *Fuse.education.vic.gov.au*. Retrieved May 12, 2021, from https://fuse.education.vic.gov.au/Resource/ByPin?Pin=X25PYT&SearchScope=All

CHAPTER 2
Why is talking about sex with children awkward?

IDENTIFYING HURDLES

For many people talking about sex and sexuality is awkward. The main reason is sex is taboo in many cultures around the world. Many people have grown up in environments where there has been a level of shame around bodies and sex, so talking about sexuality-related topics can bring up a range of emotions from awkwardness to confusion, shame and even terror. Most often these feelings get in the way of having a transparent, authentic conversation with our children and providing them with the information they need to navigate their feelings and relationships.

The first step in overcoming this barrier is to acknowledge what is happening for us. What feelings do you experience when you think about talking with your partner about sex? How about talking with your child about sex? How do you feel about talking about sex with a colleague or a manager?

My intention is not to encourage you to go share the last masturbation technique you have discovered with all your friends (although I would high-five you if you did!) but to reflect on the range of emotions you associate with sex and sexuality. What if a colleague asked you to accompany them to HR to report sexual harassment? Would you feel comfortable to sit in the meeting while the person is disclosing details of the incident? How would you feel about talking about your sexual preferences and boundaries to someone you were having sex with for the first time?

I would like to note that all 'sex talk' is not appropriate, legal or ethical. Imagine this scenario:

A man in a position of power, say a CEO, talks with a new female employee about what great sex he had the night before and how he would like to give *her* one too.

I think we would all agree that in this situation talking about sex is sexual harassment. Having a good understanding of the boundaries around who and how to share information about sexuality is important. And it is natural to have an emotional reaction when people transgress your values.

What we are trying to get to in this section is unlearning the mental/psychological programming that tells us "talking about sex under any circumstances with anyone is wrong." Or "all kind of sex is shameful, dangerous or disgusting."

Identifying mental barriers and acknowledging them is the first step towards feeling more free and at ease when it comes to sexuality-related topics.

Let's start with reflecting on the following questions:

*Important note: if you have been subjected to sexual assault as a child, the following questions may trigger strong emotions. I recommend you read them and reflect on them with a trusting friend/partner or a therapist.

Worksheet 2.1   What influenced your sexuality?

What were the messages you received from your parents about sex and sexuality? (If they never mentioned it, that is a message in itself: "we don't talk about sex in this family.")

How have these messages shaped your sexuality?

When did you first start noticing these messages?

What were the intentions of these messages?

Where did you get your first piece of sexuality information from? Was it accurate or a myth?

How did your parents/caregivers react if you touched your genitals?

How did you find out about masturbation? Did anyone talk to you about self-pleasure?

When were you first exposed to pornography?

What messages did you receive from your peers about sex when you were a teenager?

What were the messages you received from the media about sexuality?

Was your identity, sexual or otherwise, represented in these messages?

What feelings did you have about sex before your first sexual encounter?

What other complementary information did you receive as a young adult?

What are some current influences on your sexuality? (e.g. TV, media, Netflix, social media influencers, sexual health websites, family members)

Once you have identified the main messages you have received in your childhood, you can now look at them and try to identify a theme. For example, one of my clients after doing this reflective exercise discovered that two main messages from her environment had been: "Sex is dangerous" and "Men are only after what's between your legs." Although she was a well-informed and educated woman, she still associated sexuality with threat and feelings of unsafety.

Acknowledging these 'silly thoughts' and unconscious ideas can bring them up to consciousness, which allows them to be exposed to light. Denying that we have them (and we all have them) will only push them deeper into our subconscious mind where they will have more power to influence our life. Carl Jung, one of the most influential psychotherapists in history, who is best known for his theories on the human psyche, explains when we refuse to acknowledge the existence of our shadow—the unconscious part of ourselves that holds our unwanted or suppressed aspects—we deny a crucial part of our identity. As a result, these traits become magnified and inflated in our minds, and they can eventually take over our behaviour. Rejecting parts of ourselves that we find unpleasant only deepens the problem. It disconnects us from our authentic selves and leads us to believe that we are something we are not. This internal conflict can give more power to the negative traits we try to suppress, making them even more pronounced in our lives (Jung, 1984).

Our subconscious thoughts and beliefs can highly influence our attitude towards sexuality. Identifying them and reframing the ones which no longer serve us or are not relevant in our current context can help us overcome some of the discomfort of talking with our children about things which are important for their well-being and growth.

Spend some time on reframing your internalised sexual beliefs which not relevant to your current life/context anymore:

Foundations of sexuality education

Worksheet 2.2 Internalised sexual beliefs

Internalised sexual beliefs	Reframes
E.g. sexual people are at risk of being harmed	e.g. Sexual people can be safe and protected

We all have views, thoughts, beliefs and attitudes about sex (about anything in life for that matter). Our attitude and beliefs are determined by a combination of several factors: the messages we received in our childhood, our experiences in childhood and adolescence, education and knowledge we gained in adulthood, social media, pornography, culture, religion, social circumstances, peers and other experiences in life.

Discovering what your attitude towards sexuality is, what values are important to you and what triggers may exist along the way will equip you to be better prepared to have open and honest conversations with your young person about sex. Additionally, this journey of self-discovery will help you identify what you want, need and wish for in your own erotic life.

Worksheet 2.3 Attitude towards sex

Here is a list of some beliefs about sex and sexuality (Hendrick & Hendrick, 1987). For each statement select the response on the answer scale that indicates how much you agree or disagree with that statement. There are no right or wrong answers. You can simply use these statements as a guide to become more aware of your personal attitude towards sex.

Scale:

strongly agree   *moderately disagree*

moderately agree   *strongly disagree*

neutral

- I do not need to be committed to a person to have sex with him/her.

- Casual sex is acceptable.

- I would like to have sex with many partners.

- One-night stands are sometimes very enjoyable.

- It is okay to have ongoing sexual relationships with more than one person at a time.

- Sex as a simple exchange of favours is okay if both people agree to it.

- The best sex is with no strings attached.

- Life would have fewer problems if people could have sex more freely.

- It is possible to enjoy sex with a person and not like that person very much.

- It is okay for sex to be just good physical release.

- Birth control is part of responsible sexuality.

- A woman should share responsibility for birth control.

- A man should share responsibility for birth control.

- Sex is the closest form of communication between two people.

- A sexual encounter between two people deeply in love is the ultimate human interaction.

- At its best, sex seems to be the merging of two souls.

- Sex is a very important part of life.

- Sex is usually an intensive, almost overwhelming experience.

- Sex is best when you let yourself go and focus on your own pleasure.

- Sex is primarily the taking of pleasure from another person.

- The main purpose of sex is to enjoy oneself.

- Sex is primarily physical.

- Sex is primarily a bodily function, like eating.

Worksheet 2.4   Your relationship with pleasure

- What is your relationship with pleasure (sexual and non-sexual)?

- Do you think you inherently deserve to have pleasure? Or do you think you need to earn it?

- Do you consider sexual pleasure as a given or as nice to have?

- Are there any types of pleasure that you consider wrong?

- How often do you treat yourself to pleasure? Why?

- What other emotions do you associate with pleasure? (Relief? Guilt? Pride? Peace?)

Identifying triggers

Triggers are things that generate overwhelming emotions in us and as a result of those emotions we may behave in ways we wouldn't otherwise. Triggers are usually reminders of past (psychological) trauma. Sometimes triggers are predictable; for example, a survivor of sexual assault would know he would have flashbacks if he saw a movie containing any reference to rape. Sometimes we may not remember the events of the trauma, but those reminders can still elicit strong responses in us. Here is an example:

When Maria was asked by her nine-year-old son why he couldn't go for a sleep-over to his friend's house, she felt agitated and responded, "Because I say so." When he insisted, she blew up and told him to go to his room and "stop asking stupid questions".

Marie came to therapy to understand why she behaved in the way she did. She loved her son more than anything in the world and the last thing she wanted was to hurt him. She could see how her reaction was 'irrational' and out of proportion, but she couldn't understand why. "Suddenly I felt extremely angry. I just didn't want him to go."

After exploring things further Marie discovered that there was a connection to a history of trauma she had experienced at the age of nine. The assault had happened to her when she was staying at a family friend's house. She had never made the connection up until that moment, and realising that was a big moment of relief for her.

The reason we react in these 'irrational' and sometimes 'extreme' ways is because of how our brain is programmed for survival. When we are faced with a perceived threat, our emotional brain (the amygdala) comes online before our 'rational' brain (frontal cortex), this way we have the highest chance of survival. Imagine you are walking in the woods and you suddenly see a snake in the middle of the road. Most likely you will either grab something quickly to kill it (fight) or prepare to run away (flight) or you will stop and become immobile (freeze). In any case your heartbeat raises, your breathing becomes shallow, your muscles tense up and your pupils widen. After a few seconds you realise it is not a snake at all. It is just a piece of tree skin which resembles a snake. You breathe out and continue your journey. The reason our emotional brain responds first is to activate our survival responses in the body. Imagine if the rational brain came online first, if we wanted to contemplate on every situation for a few minutes or even seconds to make a decision whether it was a real threat or what the best course of action was we would have a much smaller chance of survival in the world.

So, in Marie's case, her son's age and the context (sleepover party) reminded her of a past history of a traumatic event and her emotional brain interpreted that as a threat. So, before she had the chance to rationalise it and think if it is a good idea or not, her emotional brain took control and commanded a series of behaviours to ensure Marie's offspring's survival. It may be interesting for you to know that our brain prioritises the survival of our children over our own because this means our genes will continue in the future.

But how can you identify triggers and what can you do about them? You can start by reflecting on the following questions:

Worksheet 2.5   Identifying triggers

Are there any topics related to sex that are 'off limits' for you?

Are there any topics that elicit strong emotions in you (e.g. anger, disgust, sadness, fear)?

Are there any situations in which you behave 'over the top'?

Overcoming hurdles

Planning for potential triggers

After identifying the triggers, you can do a couple of things. First, you can work with a therapist to resolve them. Although an emotional response to triggers is our brain's attempt to survive, most often they are reminders of past events and therefore are not relevant anymore. We have survived those threatening and traumatic situations, but our brain is 'stuck' in those moments. One of the most powerful ways of resolving trauma is through body-oriented psychotherapy (e.g. sensorimotor psychotherapy, somatic experiencing, Hakomi). These approaches can resolve traumatic events that we do not remember and therefore are not able to talk about.

Another thing you can do is to make a notice of the themes and situations and try to make plans around them. For example, in the context of sexuality education, if you identify topics that are emotionally charged, you can provide your child with books about those topics instead of talking about them directly or refer them to reliable sources of information on the internet. You can refer your child to another trusted adult (a partner, friend or teacher). You can have an honest conversation with your young person about why you are referring them to someone else. Something like:

> Talking about sexual assault is difficult for me. I get very emotional, but I want you to understand what it is and what to do if you ever need help. I have asked Auntie Soha to talk with you about it. Is that okay with you?

Asking your child permission to choose the source of information can be a great opportunity to teach them that they have agency and are in control of their own learning.

The rehearsal

If some topics are just uncomfortable and not triggers then practising talking about them can be a great way of overcoming the awkwardness. One of my clients found it difficult to talk about the genitalia or even to say them out loud. After practising saying them out loud when washing the dishes, in the car or in front of the mirror, she tried saying them to her partner (in the past she would only say 'down there'). These rehearsals made her much more comfortable to talk about sex and sexuality with her daughter.

Have fun with it. It doesn't have to be a dry, serious 'talk'. The more lightness you can bring to the conversation the more enjoyable and productive it can be for you and your child. Otherwise, if it turns into a formal lecture, the chances are they will zone out or use any opportunity to leave the scene.

Identifying values

Another step in overcoming discomfort is identifying what values and messages you want to communicate with your child. What are your personal values related to sexuality? Many people name mutual respect, safety and pleasure as the main values they want their children to take on board. Identifying your values can help you anchor yourself and not get lost in the details about STIs, pregnancy or gender identity, as an example. If you feel confused at times as to how to respond to a question or how to react to a situation, remind yourself of your top three values related to sexuality. Think about how you can respond within the framework of these principles.

As an example, one of my clients, Nadia, a single mother, identified mutual respect as her top value related to sexuality. When her 14-year-old daughter Svetlana asked her how she had gotten pregnant, Nadia tried to respond to the question by anchoring herself to 'mutual respect' in this way:

> Your father and I were high school sweethearts. We loved each other and went out for about a year. Back then we didn't have a good understanding of the chances of getting

pregnant if not using condoms all the time, so we wouldn't use them consistently. One day I found out I was pregnant. Although your father thought it was not the right time to have a baby, because we were in the final year of high school, he respected my decision to continue with the pregnancy. I am so glad I did, and I am so pleased we were both respectful of each other although our thoughts about the situation were very different.

Lena, another client of mine, is a mother of two children, a 10-year-old daughter and a 12-year-old son. Lena identified that she values open communication, respect and safety when it comes to sexuality. One day, her daughter asked her about periods, and Lena said she was unsure about how to respond. However, she reminded herself of her values and responded in this way:

> Sweetie, periods are a normal part of a woman's reproductive cycle. Every month, a woman's body prepares for the possibility of pregnancy, and if pregnancy doesn't happen, the body sheds the lining of the uterus, which is what we call a period. This can be uncomfortable for some women. It's important to remember to respect your body and take care of yourself during this time. You may need some extra rest. If you ever have any questions or concerns about your period or anything else related to your body, feel free to come to me and we can talk about it together.

Acknowledge discomfort

Our aim in providing sexuality education to our kids is to talk openly and honestly about any topic that comes up or is relevant. So, acknowledging our feelings about the topic is part of the process. It is completely okay to acknowledge discomfort and awkwardness when talking about sex and sexuality. You can say something like:

> I feel awkward talking about sex with you, but I think it is important and I want you to have accurate information and to know you can always come to me to ask questions although it may feel a bit awkward.

By being transparent you are role modelling vulnerability, which is one of the foundations of a happy and fulfilling (sex) life. It also creates connection and an open pathway for your child to approach you when faced with uncomfortable and confusing situations.

SELF-COMPASSION AND SELF-CARE

The path of parenthood can be rocky at times. Having doubts about yourself, your skills and what you share with your child is a common experience. Self-compassion is the fundament of coming out of the experience sane! Otherwise, we could drive ourselves and loved ones nuts!

Self-compassion is not vanity. Some parents worry that dedicating a few minutes to themselves each day for self-care would mean being lazy, self-centred and not being a good role model for their kids. On the contrary, research shows self-compassion is an antidote to self-pity and destructive self-talks. Self-compassion helps us cope with difficult situations, keeps us motivated and helps us be more supportive and caring in our relationships (Neff, 2021). When our needs are chronically unmet, we can end up feeling resentful towards our loved ones or experience moments of 'mum/dad rage'.

Self-compassion is a perspective. It means, when faced with a difficult situation and making mistakes, treating yourself with the same kindness and consideration that you would offer a good friend. Research show parents who are high on self-care and self-compassion tend to be low on self-criticism. Parents higher on self-care have better physical and mental health, whereas parents high on self-criticism tend to have poorer physical and mental health. How parents treat themselves and prioritise their own well-being has a significant impact on their child's growth and development (Giallo et al., 2015; Nelson et al., 2016; Smith & Enright, 2017). Parents who practise self-compassion and engage in self-care activities have improved health and overall wellness, are more confident in their parenting abilities and have more positive interactions with their children (Emerging Minds, 2021).

In another research high self-care and low self-criticism were also associated with reduced fatigue in parents, which result in better parenting outcomes for children (Chau & Giallo, 2015).

"But I don't have time to nurture myself" is a common complaint of busy parents. How would you respond to someone driving on an empty tank, saying "I am too busy driving I can't stop to fuel up." Self-care is not necessarily taking half a day off to go to a spa and get a full-body massage (although it could be that, too). Spending a few minutes each day to do something that *you* enjoy and doing it with mindfulness (your full attention) can do wonders.

One of the things I personally love doing is brewing tea in my special teapot and then pouring it mindfully, watching the beautiful colour stretch from the mouth of the teapot to the gorgeously patterned cup, breathing in the aroma of the freshly brewed tea and just watching the tea dancing around the cup for a few moments. The highlight for me is when I add a dash of milk and witness the delicate mushroom-like clouds that swirl in the centre of the cup. I cradle the cup in both hands, feeling the warmth seep through my fingers, and take a slow sip of the delicious tea, enjoying its luxurious flavour and richness. This ritual takes a mere ten minutes, yet it allows me to ground myself in the present and savour the serenity of the moment. It is a simple yet powerful reminder to take a moment for myself and indulge in something that brings me joy.

What are some of your favourite activities you can incorporate in your everyday life for self-care?

Here are some suggestions from parents. Each of these activities takes 5–10 minutes.

- "A few minutes of listening to my favourite music and drifting away."
- "Going for a ten-minute walk and watching the trees."
- "Dancing to my favourite song."
- "Hugging my partner without the kids being present."

- "Five extra minutes in the shower to enjoy the hot water relaxing my muscles."
- "Walking barefoot on the grass."
- "Writing in my journal. Venting."
- "Doodling while listening to music."
- "Taking a power nap."
- "Stretching my whole body."
- "Drinking a cup of coffee in silence."
- "Savouring my food."

If you want to know how to deal with the feelings of guilt when it comes to self-care or managing your child's response to you wanting to take some time off I highly recommend reading Dr. Becky Kennedy's book *Good Inside*. She has some very practical strategies to manage these sometimes difficult emotions.

PARENTS' Q&A

Table 2.1

Parent's question	My response
What do I do when I find my four-year old playing doctor or showing other kids his genitals?	Curiosity about other people's bodies and genitals is a developmentally typical behaviour in this age. Provide them books about bodies and acknowledge that it is okay to be curious and that you can help them by reading them a book.
I think that my teenage daughter might be attracted to girls, but she hasn't said anything to me. Should I ask her?	It's important to let young people take the lead about what they choose to tell you. Your child will talk to you about their sexuality when the time is right for them. The most helpful thing you can do is to create an environment where your child knows they will be supported no matter who they are. Challenge any negative statements you hear about gender and/or sexual identity of other people and proactively make it clear you are okay with gender and/or sexual diversity.
How would I answer: "How do snakes have sex?"	You can say something like: "That's an interesting question! I have no idea, but there are some great books on snakes in the library and we can see if they have the answer."

(Continued)

Table 2.1 Continued

Parent's question	My response
I believe sex is only acceptable within marriage. How can I teach my child our family's values related to sex?	One of the questions I get from many parents is: "If I believe having sex is only acceptable within marriage or a long-term relationship, can I teach my child my values around this or do I have to go with what is the latest 'trend' in society to be accepted/trusted by my child?" Teaching our kids values, our values, not only is important but mandatory as parents. It is our responsibility to teach our children values that we believe will be helpful for them in their life. Regardless of what our values are related to sexuality, we all hold values. Whether they are 'traditional' values or 'progressive', they are values. But it is important to understand that values are not static and can shift and change throughout one's life. Therefore, it is important to examine our values before imposing them on anyone, including our kids. This is the reason I have included a whole reflective section in the book about values and attitudes towards sexuality. Once we become aware of them and make a conscious and informed decision which beliefs and values are at our services, then teaching them to our children is the next step. Now to answer the question if you can tell your child that sex is only acceptable within the construct of marriage or a long-term relationship. If you have taken the steps to have a look at these beliefs and values and feel confident that they are what will lead your child to have a satisfying and fulfilling sex and romantic life, then sure, share them with your child. However, don't stop with just this small piece of information. A young person should be able to answer yes to all of these questions to make a decision whether they are ready to have sex (including within a marriage): • I know how to prevent a pregnancy from happening. • I know how to protect myself and my partner/s from STIs. You would be surprised how many people (including adults) I have met who thought a contraceptive pill could also protect them from STIs. Never assume what your child knows. • I know how to appropriately use contraception. Many people know condoms can protect them from most STIs and unintended pregnancy, but what most people don't know is HOW to correctly use a condom. For example, rolling on the condom in the correct direction is an important step. If you place the condom on the wrong way, then turn it around and reuse it, it will not fully protect you from STIs or unintended pregnancy. • I feel comfortable and safe with my partner. • I feel I could say no and that would be okay with my partner. • Nobody is forcing me to do it. • I am not forcing or pressuring my partner to do it. • I am not doing it to keep my partner.

Parent's question	My response
	• I am not doing it to make myself popular or to gain acceptance. • I feel emotionally and physically ready. • I have a pleasant feeling about the experience. And finally you can add: • I am married or in a long-term relationship. (HealthyWA, 2013) As you can see there is a lot of information our young person needs to know before deciding whether they feel ready or not. The structure of the relationship is only one point of many.

REFERENCE LIST

Chau, V., & Giallo, R. (2015). The relationship between parental fatigue, parenting self-efficacy and behaviour: Implications for supporting parents in the early parenting period. *Child: Care Health and Development*, 41(4), 626–633. https://doi.org/10.1111/cch.12221

Emerging Minds. (2021). *Parental self-care and self-compassion*. https://emergingminds.com.au/resources/parental-self-care-and-self-compassion/

Giallo, R., Treyvaud, K., Matthews, J., & Kienhuis, M. (2015). The association between parenting, child temperament, and early social-emotional development: A longitudinal study. *Infant Behavior and Development*, 38, 101–111.

HealthyWA. (2013). *Talk soon. Talk often*. Department of Health, Government of Western Australia. https://www.healthywa.wa.gov.au/~/media/HWA/Documents/Healthy-living/Sexual-health/talk-soon-talk-often.pdf

Hendrick, C., & Hendrick, S. S. (1987). The brief sexual attitudes scale. *Journal of Sex Research*, 23(3), 207–216.

Jung, C. (1984). *Dream analysis: Notes of the seminar given in 1928–1930*. Princeton University Press.

Neff, K. (2021). Self-compassion research by Kristin Neff. *Self-Compassion*. Retrieved May 28, 2021, from https://self-compassion.org/the-research/

Nelson, S. K., Kushlev, K., Lyubomirsky, S., & Gollwitzer, P. M. (2016). Putting the 'care' back in self-care: Prioritizing health and well-being as a strategy to enhance caregiving. *Journal of Social and Personal Relationships*, 33(5), 719–736.

Smith, L. E., & Enright, R. D. (2017). Parental self-forgiveness and self-compassion in parents of children with developmental disabilities. *Journal of Developmental and Physical Disabilities*, 29(1), 1–13.

CHAPTER 3
Foundations of sexuality education

Most people have had very limited sexuality and relationship education. Did you ever have a class in high school or university where you learnt how to recognise your emotions, how to articulate them to others, how to ask and give consent?

As adults most of us have had experiences of agony and joy in relationships (romantic or otherwise). Healthy sexuality doesn't mean our kids will never experience discomfort or won't make mistakes. Of course they will. This is part of being a human. But looking back when you were going through those difficult times, were there any supportive adults who provided guidance, emotional support, and helped you make sense of your experiences and decisions during those times? This is the same kind of support we aim to offer our children, providing a safe space for them to process difficult emotions, discuss their experiences and learn from any mistakes they make.

Most of us learn our sexuality and relationship education from the media, in particular Hollywood, which portrays love as easy romance. But in reality, healthy and functioning relationships require emotional intelligence skills, communication and negotiation skills and self-awareness. This is what I am attempting in this chapter: to give you some tools and techniques to teach your young ones about these essential skills. In addition, we will have a look at critical thinking skills and research skills to equip them to make well-informed decisions for their life. All these skills are transferable to other areas of life. For example, once I learnt about emotional intelligence skills I was able to negotiate much better with my colleagues, staff and family members.

I could see their point of view and utilise empathy and active listening skills to come to a point which was beneficial for both parties.

SEX EDUCATION IS MAINLY ABOUT NON-SEX STUFF!

Oscar Wilde said: "Everything in this world is about sex. Except sex, that is about power." My experience in clinical work and my research shows me that sex is never just about sex. Sex is almost always about other things, such as power, intimacy, acceptance, love, connection, a sense of well-being, control, belonging, agency, self-validation and much more.

Most of us have not been taught about honest and effective ways of communication, and therefore we may use sex to work out power dynamics in our relationships, covertly. Navigating power dynamics in a relationship, both in and out of the bedroom, can be very challenging if you don't have the right tools. For some people, the fear of rejection is so strong that they avoid initiating intimacy altogether, which includes more than just sexual acts. But as our sense of self becomes stronger and we learn to communicate effectively we can ask for what we want without taking things personally.

Sex has the potential to be much more than managing power dynamics or a rush of feel-good hormones or a sense of release. Sex can be a vehicle for deep connection, for a sense of expansion and well-being. When we learn how to open up our heart, how to be vulnerable and communicate effectively, we take sex to a completely different level.

Being able to practise vulnerability alongside some emotional intelligence skills can transform your relationships (not just the sexual and romantic ones).

TRUST (MUTUAL TRUST)

A respectful and trusting relationship with your child is the cornerstone of any interaction and of effective communication. It may be silly to point out, but sometimes in the midst of everything that is going on around us we may forget that forcing our child to sit down to have 'the talk' when they don't want to or are not ready is going to have the opposite effect of what we intend.

Coming to terms that our children are separate entities from us is hard for many of us, but it's an inevitable part of life. Children have the right to their body and life and, like everybody else, are entitled to the right to make mistakes! The concept of dignity of risk was something I learnt in my journey as a mental health practitioner. Dignity of risk means people regardless of their age should have the freedom to make decisions and choices that may expose them to a level of risk. In other words, we all have the fundamental right to make mistakes and learn and grow from trial and error. Dignity of risk as opposed to over-protection provides people with an opportunity for personal growth.

Positive risk-taking can lead to:

- improved autonomy
- improved social interaction
- improved health
- opportunity for living independently
- constructing one's life in accordance with their values and personality
- self-determination and feelings of worth

Over-protection can lead to

- feeling patronised
- feeling smothered
- loss of hope
- feeling diminished
- preventing individuals from reaching their potentials
- preventing individuals from learning from their mistakes

I would like to note that dignity of risk does not eliminate our responsibility as parents to care for our children's wellbeing. Duty of care could mean providing options and reasonable level of information for our children to make age-appropriate decisions.

This perspective to education and parenting helps us move away from smothering our kids and inadvertently pushing them further away from us. It also sends the message to young people that they need to make sound, responsible decisions for their lives. It also facilitates an environment of mutual trust where, when they are in doubt, they can always approach us or in our absence select a suitable substitute.

A NOTE ON SHAME

Children's behaviours are driven by their need for survival, and their resources are dependent on their parents or caregivers. Therefore, they often exhibit behaviours that maximise their connection with their caregiver as a survival strategy. When children feel shame, they may hide things from their parents to protect themselves and maximise their survival chances.

It's important for us as parents to understand the function of shame and how it impacts our children's behaviour. Shaming our children for touching their genitals or asking sexuality-related questions may push them away from us, creating a distance in the relationship. When children feel disconnected from their parents, they may seek validation and resources from other sources, which may not be safe or reliable.

Therefore, it's essential to create a safe and supportive home environment for children to explore their sexuality and ask questions. When caregivers shame children, they may inadvertently teach them to feel ashamed of their bodies and sexuality, which can lead to long-term negative impacts on their relational, sexual and mental health.

As you read this book, you may encounter feelings of shame related to your own experiences with sexuality or parenting. It's important to approach these feelings with gentleness and compassion, recognising that at some point in your life, shame protected you and maximised your survival chances. By being compassionate with yourself, you may relate to the feelings of shame with greater understanding and empathy, allowing yourself to experience other emotions such as curiosity, and enthusiasm for learning.

Sexuality-related topics are often surrounded by stigma and shame, making it difficult for many people to discuss these topics openly. This stigma can lead to confusion, fear, and a lack of understanding in children. As a parent, creating a safe environment at home and destigmatising sexuality can help your child feel more comfortable discussing these topics. When having conversations about sexuality, use this formula: "De-shame + Connect" (Kennedy, 2022).

De-shaming means removing the negative associations surrounding sexuality-related topics. Connecting means creating an environment where your child feels comfortable asking questions and discussing their thoughts and feelings. You can let them know that you are always available to talk about sex-related topics and that you are open to learning alongside them. For example, if you catch your 13-year-old watching porn, you can say something like this: "I saw you were watching porn on your laptop. It is normal and healthy to be curious about sex" (de-shame). "Porn is only for adults. If you have any questions about sex, I'd love to talk with you about them. If I don't know the answer we can find it out together" (connect). "If it feels tricky to talk to me, I can show you some reliable websites."

Here's another example: if your child tells you they are a different gender to what they were assigned at birth, you can use the "De-shame + Connect" formula to create a supportive and inclusive environment. You can start by letting them know that you love and support them and that their gender identity is normal and healthy. You can say something like:

> I'm proud of you for being true to yourself and for having the courage to express yourself the way it feels right.

If you ever want to talk about your feelings or experiences, I'm here to listen and support you in any way I can.

REFERENCE LIST

Kennedy, B. (2022). *Good inside: A guide to becoming a better parent.* HarperOne.

Part 2
Sexual intelligence skills

CHAPTER 4

Attachment styles and their role in adulthood relationships

Attachment theory, developed by John Bowlby and Mary Ainsworth, looks at the way our childhood experiences impact how we connect with others, especially significant others, in our adult life. According to this theory, one's relationship with their parents during childhood has an overarching influence on their social, intimate relationships and even relationships at work in the future. In other words, your early relationship with your parents and caregivers sets the stage for how you will build relationships as an adult.

WHAT DOES 'ATTACHMENT' MEAN IN THIS CONTEXT?

The emotional connection formed by emotional communication between an infant and their parent or primary caregiver is known as attachment (Healthline, 2021).

THE STRANGE SITUATION

In 1969 psychologist Mary Ainsworth and her colleagues ran experiments known as The Strange Situation, which observed and identified attachment behaviours in children. (You can watch this interesting—but somewhat upsetting—experiment on YouTube.) The researchers brought mothers and their babies into the lab and had them play in a room with toys on the floor and with other adults coming in and out of the room. At some point, the mothers would leave the room for a few minutes, leaving the child behind. After a while, they'd return. The aim of the research was to observe how children responded first to their caregiver leaving and later to their caregiver returning to them.

Here are some of the patterns they observed (Smith et al., 1970):

- Some babies explored and played freely when their mother was in the room, became distressed when she left and then calmed down upon her return. These children were labelled as securely attached.
- Some children avoided or ignored their mothers even before she left and showed little emotion when left in the room and when she returned. Ainsworth and her colleagues hypothesised that this avoidant behaviour masked their true distress, and some further research tracking their heart rates confirmed this theory. Although on the surface these children looked placid, their heart rate showed they experienced the same level of distress as the securely attached children. These children were labelled as avoidant.
- Some children showed distress before the mother left, got significantly more distressed when she did, and were hard to comfort when she returned. They continued to cry and show distress despite the fact that the mother had returned and was trying to soothe them. These children were labelled as anxious.
- Finally, some children showed largely inconsistent behaviours, including disorganisation or disorientation in the form of wandering, confused expressions, freezing, undirected movements, fear of the caregiver or even aggression towards them. Sometimes they'd have these moments of out-of-place behaviours and then fall into one of the other categories, or they would be a mix of several. These children were labelled as having disorganised attachment.

HOW DO ATTACHMENT STYLES DEVELOP IN EARLY CHILDHOOD?

Whether your parents respond to your emotional needs consistently has a lasting impact on our relational patterns and how we form relationships later in life.

As babies and young children, we are dependent on our caregivers and seek comfort, soothing and support from them. If our physical and emotional needs are satisfied, we form a secure attachment style. This, however, requires that our caregivers offer a warm and caring environment and are attuned to our needs. Misattunement (not recognising and responding to the emotional needs of the child consistently) on the side of the parent, on the other hand, is likely to lead to insecure attachment in their children.

There are four attachment styles that people can have. The secure attachment style is characterised by a sense of ease and comfort with emotional closeness to others, as well as with others being emotionally close to them. People with a secure attachment style are able to trust others and be trustworthy, give and receive love and form close relationships relatively easily. They don't feel afraid of intimacy, nor do they become fearful when their partner/s express a need for time or space apart from them. They can rely on others without losing their independence (Holmes, 2011).

As individuals grow up, having a secure attachment style is associated with several positive outcomes, such as increased self-esteem, forming more healthy and lasting relationships and having a greater capacity to rely on others for social support. This is because individuals with secure attachment styles had positive experiences with their caregivers growing up, which serves as a blueprint for forming healthy bonds with others in different types of relationships, including romantic and sexual relationships (Mikulincer & Shaver, 2016).

According to foundational attachment research by social psychologists Cindy Hazan and Phillip Shaver (1987), about 56% of adults have a secure attachment style.

The other three styles are insecure attachments and are as follows (Mikulincer & Shaver, 2016):

AVOIDANT

The avoidant attachment style is a type of insecure attachment style that is characterised by a fear of intimacy. This can lead to a reluctance to get too close to others or to share personal feelings, which in turn causes people with this attachment style to become more self-reliant. Trusting others in relationships can be difficult for individuals with an avoidant attachment style, and they may feel suffocated by relationships.

Partners of individuals with an avoidant attachment style may desire more intimacy in their relationship, both sexually and emotionally. However, individuals with this attachment style may prioritise physical sensations over emotional connections, and activities such as cuddling or gazing into each other's eyes may feel too vulnerable.

ANXIOUS

The anxious attachment style is an insecure attachment style characterised by a strong fear of abandonment. Individuals with this style of attachment desire intimacy but also fear being alone. They often feel insecure about their relationships, constantly seeking validation and worrying that their partner will leave them. Behaviours associated with this attachment style include being overly needy and clingy, getting anxious when their partner wants alone time and feeling like their partner doesn't care enough. Additionally, people with an anxious attachment style may prioritise their partner's sexual desires over their own.

DISORGANISED ATTACHMENT

This attachment style comes from traumatic or abusive experiences during childhood. Because of this, positive feelings of love and affection can be closely tied to feelings of fear and danger.

People with a fearful-avoidant attachment style both want and fear closeness with others. They may avoid developing close romantic relationships but still crave intimacy and affection. They might have intense positive feelings towards someone and then distance themselves for a while afterwards. In sexual relationships, they may feel disconnected from their body or may find their experiences of sex unpredictable.

HOW EACH ATTACHMENT STYLE IS FORMED

Our attachment styles are usually formed during early childhood and are shaped by our interactions with our primary caregivers. The way caregivers respond to a child's emotional distress cues is a significant factor in determining their attachment style (Mikulincer & Shaver, 2016).

"Human beings are born helpless, so we are hardwired at birth to search for and attach to a reliable caregiver for protection," Peter Lovenheim, author of *The Attachment Effect*, says. "The quality of that first bond—loving and stable or inconsistent or even absent—actually shapes the developing brain, influencing us throughout life in how we deal with loss and how we behave in relationships" (Sosa, 2020).

Here is a summary of what circumstances lead to each of the four attachment types:

SECURE ATTACHMENT

Children who are securely attached feel safe and have someone they can trust. They show a preference for their caregiver over strangers, seek comfort from their caregiver and feel at ease exploring their surroundings when their caregiver is present. Caregivers of securely attached children are attentive to their child's physical and emotional needs and respond with care and empathy. For instance, when a child is upset, they try to comfort and understand their distress.

A secure attachment has three characteristics (Bretherton & Munholland, 2008):

- Provides a sense of safety and security.
- Regulates emotions by soothing distress and supporting calm.
- Offers a secure base from which to explore.

You may find it comforting to know that even when parents are attuned to the needs of the child only 30% of the time, the child can develop a secure attachment style (Bowlby, 1987).

AVOIDANT ATTACHMENT

Children who develop an avoidant attachment style tend to avoid their caregivers and do not seek comfort from them. They show little to no preference for their caregiver over a stranger, and do not reach out to their parents when they need help. This attachment style typically forms when parents or caregivers are emotionally unavailable or unresponsive to the child's needs. As a result, the child learns that they cannot rely on their caregiver for comfort and care, and may even see a stranger as a better source of support (Mikulincer & Shaver, 2016).

ANXIOUS ATTACHMENT

The inconsistency of caregivers' emotional responses, including being overly involved or withdrawn, leads children to develop an anxious attachment. These children may cling to their caregiver and avoid exploring or playing in their presence. When the caregiver leaves, children with an anxious attachment become distressed, and upon their return they may exhibit a combination of clinginess and angry reactions such as struggling, hitting or pushing back (Mikulincer & Shaver, 2016).

DISORGANISED ATTACHMENT

This attachment style can develop in families where the child is exposed to abuse or neglect from their caregiver, who is meant to be a source of comfort and safety. The caregiver may be directly causing harm to the child, or they may have their own history of trauma that has not been resolved (Mikulincer & Shaver, 2016).

HOW TO PARENT FOR A SECURE ATTACHMENT

As caregivers we need to be involved, attentive, sensitive and responsive. Children, even infants, communicate with us all the time. Pay attention to what they are trying to communicate, get curious about their internal state. Your child will tell you what to do. Babies and young children have a limited way of expressing their needs, so they are not that difficult to read: If they are crying, they need something. If their arms are out, they want to be picked up. And if you misread them, don't stress, they will keep on signalling until you get it right.

One of the resources for how to parent for a secure attachment in the first few years of life is the book *Raising a Secure Child* by Kent Hoffman, Glen Cooper and Bert Powell. The authors are therapists who have worked with many families and children over the years. They emphasise the importance of attachment and call their approach the 'Circle of Security'. According to the authors, parenting for secure attachment is not a set of specific behaviours, but rather a state of mind, where parents are sensitive to their child's feelings and needs. The book also helps parents identify their own attachment style and make any necessary changes to promote secure attachment with their child (Hoffman, 2017). Another great resource is Fr Becky Kennedy's book *Good Inside*. She has some very practical strategies to responding to tricky situations and fostering a secure attachment with children.

Some things to consider about the attachment theory:

- Attachment theory is based on a 'Western' understanding of self and culture. It does not take into account parenting in collective cultures where children are parented by many attachment figures and they don't develop a bond with one person or with their biological parents but with the whole community. In many cultures which have multiple caregivers, the child doesn't have separation anxiety and they don't have a fear of strangers (Ogden et al., 2019).
- Early childhood attachment with a parent is not destiny. Through a 'corrective emotional experience', which involves feeling safe with someone who meets our needs and accepts us for who we are, we can heal our attachment style in adulthood. This can also occur with the guidance of a therapist, as the therapeutic process mirrors the attachment process. By healing attachment ruptures, we can form more secure relationship patterns.
- Attachment is a complex topic, and if looked at superficially it can make us feel we are either secure or have a 'messed up' attachment. The truth is, attachment is much more complex and nuanced than how we've been understanding it. So use this framework as a guide to understand the importance of early childhood attunement with your children but not a tool for diagnosis.

REFERENCE LIST

Bowlby, J. (1987). The role of attachment in personality development and psychopathology. In N. Feather (Ed.), *The psychobiology of personality* (pp. 51–67). Springer. https://doi.org/10.1007/978-1-4684-4758-2_4

Bretherton, I., & Munholland, K. A. (2008). Internal working models in attachment relationships: A construct revisited. In J. Cassidy & P. R. Shaver (Eds.), *Handbook of attachment: Theory, research, and clinical applications* (pp. 102–127). Guilford Press.

Hazan, C., & Shaver, P. (1987). Romantic love conceptualized as an attachment process. *Journal of Personality and Social Psychology,*

52(3), 511–524. https://www2.psych.ubc.ca/~schaller/Psyc591Readings/HazanShaver1987.pdf

Healthline. (2021, May 27). What is secure attachment and how can you cultivate it? *Healthline*. Retrieved March 31, 2023, from https://www.healthline.com/health/secure-attachment-2

Hoffman, B. (2017). *Raising a secure child: How circle of security parenting can help you nurture your child's attachment, emotional resilience, and freedom to explore*. Guilford Press.

Holmes, J. G. (2011). Attachment, intimacy, and close relationships. In S. J. Lopez & C. R. Snyder (Eds.), *The Oxford handbook of positive psychology* (2nd ed., pp. 393–401). Oxford University Press.

Mikulincer, M., & Shaver, P. R. (2016). *Attachment in adulthood: Structure, dynamics, and change* (2nd ed.). Guilford Press.

Ogden, P., Fisher, J., & Pain, C. (2019). *Pocket guide to sensorimotor psychotherapy*. W. W. Norton & Company.

Smith, J. D., Terry, D. J., Manstead, A. S. R., Louis, W. R., Kotterman, D., & Wolfs, J. (1970). Attributional confidence and social perception: The case of actors' versus observers' perceptions of causality. *European Journal of Social Psychology*, 1(4), 385–399. https://doi.org/10.1002/ejsp.2420010402

Sosa, T. (2020). *The attachment effect: Exploring the powerful ways our earliest bond shapes our relationships and lives*. Penguin Books.

CHAPTER 5
Emotional intelligence skills

Reflect on the following statements. Which one do you agree with (Matthews et al., 2012, p. 105)?

Passionate emotions are dangerous, causing people to act foolishly in fits of anger and exuberance.

Emotions are critical for providing motivation, purpose and meaning in everyday life.

Do you prefer to make decisions by logic or emotion? Why?

Parents' responses to their children's emotions are influenced by their underlying beliefs about emotions. Sometimes, when children express strong emotions, parents may try to take control instead of trying to understand their child's feelings. As parents want to shield their children, they may find it difficult to be honest about their own emotions, or they may avoid discussing the topic altogether.

When parents react negatively to their children's emotions, children can start to believe that emotions are negative and something to be avoided or hidden. This can lead to difficulty managing and expressing emotions later in life. It's important for parents to teach their children that emotions are a normal and healthy part of being human and that there are ways to manage them effectively. By doing so, children can learn to understand and work through their emotions in a healthy way.

Emotional intelligence is the ability to identify and regulate one's emotions and understand the emotions of the others. A high level of emotional intelligence helps you to build relationships, reduce stress, defuse conflict and improve your sense of satisfaction (La Trobe University, 2021).

Research (Cotrus et al., 2012) shows more than IQ, emotional intelligence (EQ) seems to determine success in life. The ability to understand other people and work with them is critical to success in modern work life. It is also critical in relationships, and we know that having successful friendships and romantic and sexual relationships results in enormous benefits in health, wealth, happiness and longevity (Gottman, 2018).

A study discovered that there are two distinct parenting styles when it comes to managing emotions and emotional intelligence. Emotion dismissing parents tend to be action-oriented and avoid emotional engagement as they view emotions as potentially harmful. On the other hand, emotion coaching parents accept and explore emotions in themselves and others. The research revealed that the effects of these approaches were significant, with children of the two types of parents experiencing different outcomes in life. In the case of divorced families, emotion coaching was found to buffer children from most of the negative effects of their parents' divorce. As a result, two children with the same IQ at age four could have vastly different educational achievements by age eight (Gottman, 2018)!

Due to the limited scope of this book, I cannot provide an extensive discussion on emotional intelligence. But I'll give you a quick overview of the main elements, so you can get an idea of what it's all about. If you want to learn more, there are plenty of books and articles out there that go into more detail.

HOW DOES EMOTIONAL INTELLIGENCE RELATE TO SEXUALITY?

Emotional intelligence can have a significant impact on sexual relationships and sexual health outcomes. People with higher emotional intelligence are better equipped to communicate effectively, understand their own emotions and the emotions of their partner and empathise with their partner's needs and desires. This can lead to more satisfying and fulfilling sexual experiences for both partners. Additionally, emotional intelligence can help individuals make informed decisions about their sexual health, communicate their boundaries and needs and navigate complex situations, such as consent and safer sex practices.

Here are some examples of how emotional intelligence can relate to successful sexual relationships and better sexual health outcomes:

- Communication: Emotional intelligence can help individuals communicate their needs, desires and boundaries effectively. For example, someone with high emotional intelligence may be able to clearly express their sexual preferences and comfort level to their partner, leading to a more satisfying and enjoyable sexual experience for both parties.
- Empathy: Emotional intelligence can also help individuals understand and empathise with their partner's needs and emotions. For instance, someone with high emotional intelligence may be able to recognise when their partner is not in the mood for sex and respond with empathy, rather than pressuring or coercing them.
- Resilience: Emotional intelligence can help individuals bounce back from rejection or negative experiences, which can be especially important in the context of sexual relationships. For example, someone with high emotional intelligence may be able to handle rejection or a sexual encounter that didn't go as planned without experiencing lasting negative effects on their self-esteem or mental health.
- Self-awareness: Emotional intelligence involves being aware of one's own emotions and how they influence behaviour. This can be helpful in sexual relationships because it allows individuals to recognise when they may be acting out of negative emotions (such as jealousy or insecurity) and address those issues before they impact the relationship.

EMOTIONAL INTELLIGENCE IN PARENTING BEGINS WITH THE SELF

Emotional intelligence begins with oneself. It is important to understand our own feelings about emotions and to learn that self-understanding comes from identifying our own feelings. As John Gottman says, emotions are our internal GPS through life. The ability to recognise an emotion as we experience it is the key to emotional intelligence.

Being emotional doesn't mean being irrational. Often, there is a misconception that feelings and rational responses are in opposition. Emotions serve a function; all of them. Even the difficult ones, the ones we don't want to experience. For example, anger motivates us to address the source of something that feels threatening to us. Fear motivates us to flee and protect ourselves when faced with a threat. Jealousy acts like a compass, showing us where we need to head to feel more fulfilled. In order to understand what action to take to feel safer, happier, more fulfilled we first need to *feel* the emotions and not repress them. All emotions are welcome: anger, sadness, joy, despair, frustration, excitement, confusion, to name a few. By recognising them and labelling them we can then take the next step to understand them.

Many people have grown up in environments where feeling a certain type of emotion was looked down upon. In a generalised way, male-identifying people are often raised not to show sadness, despair and vulnerability, and female-identifying people are often told to repress anger and desire.

So, many of us supress these emotions and hide them away in our subconscious. It is surprising for many of my male clients to discover that the constant rage they experience is actually fear or sadness.

As children we cannot risk losing the support or love of our caregivers, and we certainly cannot ask for different ones, but what we can do is adjust our behaviour and our emotions to maximise the support and resources we receive from them. However, when these emotions are repressed for a very long time and not expressed, they can influence our life from the deep corners of our subconscious and surprise us with unintended behaviours.

Worksheet 5.1   Identifying emotions

Take a few moments and reflect on the following questions:

What emotions were taboo in my family of origin?

What type of feelings did I feel I had to hide or tone down?

How do I feel those emotions now?

How do I express them now?

Salovey and Mayer's four-branch model of emotional intelligence suggests that we need to nurture and develop four abilities to deal with the emotional content of our lives: perceiving emotions (emotional literacy), facilitating emotions, understanding emotions and managing emotions (Watkins & Huang, 2003).

The first is the ability to perceive our emotions. This is the basic component of emotional intelligence. Being able to accurately identify and label emotions in ourselves and others is the first step. As an example, being able to pick up on non-verbal cues too, such as reading the body language of your child when the verbal and non-verbal messages don't match or recognising when you (or your child) are getting angry and expressing your emotions appropriately.

Secondly, we need to understand what to do with emotions once they have been recognised. This includes remaining grounded and resilient in the face of challenging situations and being able to overcome emotional challenges, such as conflicts with family members or co-workers, by using helpful behaviours and responses.

Next is understanding emotions. In other words, the ability to recognise the subtle differences between emotional states, such as the difference between hate and dislike or that some emotions might be made up of multiple components. For example, contempt could be made up of disgust and anger. It also refers to the understanding of how emotions can be transitional. So, for example, speaking angrily to your child may lead to regret subsequently (Mayer et al., 2004).

EMOTIONAL LITERACY

Before getting emotionally intelligent we need to be emotionally literate. Emotional literacy in basic terms means the ability to pause and asking ourselves "what am I feeling?" and have an answer. For example, some people might get angry to disguise their feelings of insecurity, and some might act like they're having a great time at a party even if they're really feeling sad inside.

For many people *feeling* can get confused with *thinking*. Here is what I mean: In couple therapy sessions I often ask one of the partners how he/she feels about the situation, and they respond with: "I feel my partner is wrong!" They are surprised when I say: "that is what you are thinking. What are you *feeling*?" and on many occasions I see a blank look on their face.

Since many of us have never been taught to identify and recognise feelings it can take time to learn this skill. How many of us had a teacher at school ask us, "how are you feeling right now? Not thinking, feeling."

So here are some steps to take to identify emotions and feelings and distinguish them from thoughts. As a rule of thumb if feeling is followed by 'that' it is usually a thought and not a feeling. For example, the following statements are thoughts:

> "I feel that I need more space."
> "I feel I am being manipulated by you."
> "I feel we would make a great couple."

Emotional intelligence skills

Worksheet 5.2   Exploring and identifying emotions

How many of these emotions have you experienced in the last seven days? You can set an intention to get curious about your feelings and emotional state by paying attention to what new emotions you experience (or notice) in the next seven days. Take some notes.

Happiness	Disappointment	Disgust
Sadness	Frustration	Pride
Anger	Boredom	Shame
Love	Elation	Guilt
Fear	Loneliness	Anticipation
Anxiety	Empathy	Curiosity
Jealousy	Sympathy	Awe
Envy	Gratitude	Confusion
Excitement		

SELF-MANAGEMENT

The next step after identifying emotions and becoming aware of the underlying ones, is to learn how to regulate them. Most often our first reaction is wanting to get rid of them. However, more and more research (Heydari et al., 2018) shows that trying to control emotions or actively trying to get rid of them can exacerbate the intensity and frequency of them. 'So, what can I do?' you ask. There are many ways to manage emotions without causing harm to ourselves and others.

One step involves naming what we are feeling. For example: "I feel scared." Just by stating that, we start to shift the process because we have accessed a different part of the brain (frontal cortex) which isn't responsible for our survival needs (mostly known as fight/flight/freeze response). The cortex interprets the bodily sensations and puts them into language. So stating or labelling your emotion is the first step of self-management (Torre & Lieberman, 2018).

The second step is understanding where a feeling is. Basically, feelings are set of vibrations or sensations in the body (usually combined with a thought but are separate from thoughts). So the second question we ask ourselves is: "where is the fear (or the emotion that you are experiencing) in the body?" Most people intuitively respond to this question, for example: "it is in my stomach, in the centre of my chest, etc."

The next question is "what are the sensations doing?" or "what are those bodily sensations?" Look for the answer in your body. You may sense heat, nausea, contraction, expansion, pulsing, etc. In a world where we are constantly bombarded by noise and external stimuli this simple step might take practice to master. It is okay if at first you can't name the sensations. Approach it with curiosity, and eventually you will discover what your body is experiencing.

The next question is: "could you place your attention on the sensations for a couple of moments?" This is the key step; this is where there will be a subtle move to give the feeling presence. Most of us don't have a healthy relationship with feelings, so when difficult emotions such as fear come up, we tend to repress them, supress them or get paralysed by them. So, ask: "could I just allow the belly to gurgle? Could I allow the heat in my face for a few moments?" and this 'permission' is what gets the energy released.

When we repress or supress the feelings they get stuck in the body. They can turn into movements and postures which can perpetuate those feelings even more. Our body is communicating with us every minute of the day. If my shoulders are hunched and I am collapsed in my body, I hear my body communicating to me that there is something scary happening and I'm not safe. That in turn creates certain thought patterns and feelings of unsafety and incompetence.

You can use the following questions to understand the sensations and the feeling on a deeper level (Ray, 2021):

- If you could trace an outline around the feeling as if it were an object, what shape would it be?
- What colour is the feeling?
- What texture does the feeling have on the inside? And what texture does it have on the outside?
- Does the feeling have a weight?
- Does the feeling have a temperature?
- Is the feeling still or moving?
- What kind of substance is the feeling made of? Air? Metal? Liquid?
- How big is the feeling? How much of your body is it taking up?

Once you identify the feeling and how it presents in the body, the final step is asking the emotion what it is here to show you.

Table 5.1 provides some examples of the most common emotions and some *possible* messages they try to communicate (Ray, 2021).

Table 5.1 Understanding common emotions and their messages

Emotion	Possible message
Fear	Something in my space (life) is or seems to be threatening.
Uncertainty	I am exploring unfamiliar territories.
Self-doubt	I am forgetting my strengths.
Withdrawn	There is something I need to process alone.
Guilt	Either I have a legitimate mistake to correct or I am dishonouring my own needs in favour of others.
Demotivation	I need a break or change of direction.
Overwhelmed	I am asking too much of myself.
Frustrated	I am blocked or stuck in some way.
Angry	A boundary of mine has been crossed.
Mistrust	I have given a piece of myself previously that has been mishandled.
Betrayal	My loyalty has been disrespected.
Jealousy	I believe I deserve the same in my life.
Grief	I have lost something precious to me.
Loneliness	I need a companion.
Disappointment	Something didn't work out as I hoped.
Rejection	My sense of belonging is shaken.
Shame	I am rejecting a part of myself.
Regret	I have learnt a difficult lesson.
Dissatisfaction	I crave discovery.
Boredom	My curiosity wants to be fed.
Unworthiness	My inner world is asking to be nurtured.
Exhaustion	My reserves are empty.

So, this is the summary of the process:

- What emotion are you feeling? Name it.
- Where is the emotion in the body?
- What is it doing? What sensations do you feel in the body?
- Could you just allow these sensations for a few moments?
- What does this feeling want you to pay attention to?

It may sound overly simplistic or even 'airy-fairy', but all the techniques I have shared are evidence-based psychological frameworks. If you are interested, look up acceptance commitment therapy and sensorimotor psychotherapy.

WHAT DOES IT LOOK LIKE IN PARENTING?

Jason, a father of two, responds to his five-year-old when she is scared in this way:

> "Sweety, you are scared. It is okay to be scared. I get scared too."
>
> And then: "Would you like me to hold you for a moment? What do you need?"

When feelings are met with acceptance they naturally release. They won't cause us all sorts of somatic problems for the rest of our lives and in our relationships. So, after we accept the feeling, we can get curious about the reason. "What are you scared of?" and then "why?"

As I said earlier all emotions have a function. For example, anger is usually inviting us to see that something is not of service to us and to make a change, for example, to put some boundaries in place.

This is a technique I teach couples to do together which produces a tremendous level of intimacy and connection. Next time your partner is feeling an emotion you can ask them: "what emotion is present?" or "what are you feeling?" And then: "can we be with it for a while?" and "where in your body are you feeling it?"

Practise this technique until you've got the hang of it. It can take some time to remember the questions to ask yourself. As with any technique that you are learning to apply in real life, this might feel clunky and 'unnatural' at first. Bu the more you practise the more you'll notice your relationship with your mind and emotions changes. So, write them down on a cue card or somewhere that they are accessible throughout the day to look at and refer to them until they come naturally to you.

Here are some evidence-based psychological frameworks that can help manage emotional distress. Next time you feel stressed or overwhelmed when your child has a tantrum or you think they are being unreasonable and difficult, try one of these techniques.

Instead of reacting impulsively, you can take a few deep breaths and use these mindfulness techniques to stay calm and centred in the moment. You can observe your own thoughts and feelings, without getting caught up in them, and tune in to your child's emotions and needs.

By practising self-regulation techniques, we can become more aware of our own emotional triggers and patterns of behaviour, which can help us respond to our children in a more compassionate and effective way. We can also model mindfulness to our children and help them develop their own emotional regulation skills.

SELF-REGULATION TECHNIQUE: SIT WITH YOURSELF (RAY, 2021)

Sometimes you don't need to do anything with your emotions other than to sit through them. How can you do that when your mind is suggesting anything but? Try some of these strategies to help you calm your nervous system in the present moment:

- Instead of judging, observe your emotions and experiences with curiosity.

Emotional intelligence skills

- Remind yourself that this too shall pass.
- Validate your emotions.
- Acknowledge the unhelpful thoughts.
- Resist the urge to push away emotional discomfort and instead allow yourself to sit with it.
- Engage in calming activities, such as taking a mindful walk or drinking tea.

SELF-REGULATION TECHNIQUE: MINDFULNESS

This simple, yet effective exercise is helpful with intense emotions such as anxiety, anger or panic attacks. By paying attention to the present moment (mindfulness) and naming sensory stimuli, we are engaging the prefrontal cortex, which is the part of the brain responsible for logical thinking, and reduce the activity in the limbic system, which is in charge of survival responses and emotions. Obviously if there is a real threat present in the environment our emotions need to be taken seriously and actions need to be taken to ensure safety.

Before starting this exercise, pay attention to your breathing. Slow, deep, long breaths can help you maintain a sense of calm or help you return to a calmer state (by activating the parasympathetic nervous system, which leads to decreased arousal).

- Name FIVE things you see around you. It could be a pen, a spot on the ceiling, anything in your surroundings.
- Name FOUR things you can touch around you. It could be your hair, a pillow or the ground under your feet.
- Name THREE things you hear. This could be any external sound. If you can hear your belly rumbling that counts!
- Name TWO things you can smell. Maybe you are in your office and smell graphite from a pencil, or maybe you are in your bedroom and smell a pillow. If you need to take a brief walk to find a scent, you could smell soap in your bathroom or scents of nature outside.
- Name ONE thing you can taste. What does the inside of your mouth taste like—gum, coffee or the sandwich from lunch?

SELF-REGULATION TECHNIQUE: SQUARE BREATHING (MAHTANI, 2020)

Square breathing, also known as box breathing, is a technique used when taking slow, deep breaths. It can heighten performance and concentration while also being a powerful stress reliever.

- Sitting upright, slowly exhale through your mouth, getting all the oxygen out of your lungs. Focus on this intention and be conscious of what you're doing.
- Inhale slowly and deeply through your nose to the count of four. In this step, count to four very slowly in your head. Feel the air fill your lungs, one section at a time, until your lungs are completely full and the air moves into your abdomen.
- Hold your breath for another slow count of four.
- Exhale through your mouth for the same slow count of four. Pay attention to the feeling of the air leaving your lungs.
- Hold your breath for the same slow count of four before repeating this process.

Repeat this process until you notice your symptoms of stress, anxiety or anger have reduced.

SELF-REGULATION TECHNIQUE: GROUND YOURSELF IN NATURE (RAY, 2021)

Step outside and into nature. Forest-bathing is effective because it has tremendous calming effects, as does being near the beach or walking in a garden. Feeling overwhelmed by emotions? Go outside.

TIPS ON RAISING EMOTIONALLY INTELLIGENT KIDS (CURTIS, 2021)

1. Take care of yourself
Parenting is one of the hardest roles in the world. Emotionally intelligent parents are compassionate towards themselves as

well as others. They understand that emphasising their own well-being will make them more patient, joyful and energetic. They acknowledge their needs are valid and invest resources in practising self-care. When they find themselves getting exhausted or overwhelmed, they take steps to course-correct and prioritise themselves.

2. Focus on connection
One of the crucial steps in emotionally intelligent parenting is establishing a deep connection with your child. In today's world, filled with distractions and noise, it is easy to lose focus and feel stressed. Connecting with your child doesn't need to take up too much time. Emotionally intelligent parents take steps to create micro-moments of connection, develop daily or weekly rituals and create special moments with their child.

3. Practise emotion coaching
Emotion coaching your child involves being aware of your child's emotions, helping them identify and label their feelings and fostering emotional regulation. Emotionally intelligent parents do not dismiss or criticise their child's emotions. Instead, they view their child's difficult feelings as opportunities to empathise, connect and teach. They empower their child to develop strategies for coping with emotionally challenging situations.

Picture this scene: You serve your child's favourite breakfast—a peanut butter sandwich—on her favourite plate at her favourite seat at the table. And what do you receive in return? A high-pitched "I HATE peanut butter sandwiches!"

"But this is your favourite breakfast. You told me so yourself!"

"NOOOO. . . ."

"But last week you ate it happily!"

"NOOOO. . . ."

It is easy to get frustrated when you can't make your child see reason! Next time a similar scenario happens consider acknowledging your child's emotions and helping them realise what they are experiencing.

So instead of saying, "You know you love peanut butter sandwiches! This is your favourite breakfast!" try: "Sounds like you're disappointed about a peanut butter sandwich for breakfast. You're in the mood for something different."

4. Set boundaries to teach, not to punish
Emotionally intelligent parents prioritise setting boundaries with their children by respectfully teaching them what is expected of them in different situations and the consequences of crossing those boundaries. They do not discipline their children as a form of punishment, but rather use consistency and support to help their children maintain healthy boundaries and limits. Yelling, ignoring or punishing may achieve short-term results, but it does not teach children the necessary skills to manage their behaviour in the long run.

5. Teach your kids about your values
Values are beliefs that individuals hold to be important for themselves and society. They influence our behaviours, attitudes and decisions, making it essential to consider them in parenting. Spend time on identifying your own values and communicating them to your children. However, keep in mind that simply telling your child to be more honest or hard-working or grateful or compassionate doesn't work any better than telling adults to be. As parents we need to model the values we uphold and label and reinforce the expression of values. Explain why you make certain decisions based on your values and encourage your child's initiatives that express their values.

CASE EXAMPLES

Manuel and Lucia
Manuel was watching a movie with his daughter, Lucia. The protagonist seemed to use emotional manipulation to get what she wanted. Manuel used this opportunity to talk with

Lucia about some values that were very important to him and his family.

Manuel: "What did you think of the way Margaret (the character in the movie) was acting?"
Lucia: "I didn't like how she was trying to make Arthur feel bad."
Manuel: "I had the same feeling. I think she was trying to stand up for what she wanted, but she did it in a way that was disrespectful of Arthur's boundaries. Honesty and fairness are really important for me."

Marcia and Dani

Marcia and Dani were at a department store when Dani asked his mum to buy an expensive toy. When Marcia said no, Dani started yelling and begging her for the toy. Marcia took one long intentional deep breath and tried to focus on the connection of her feet with the floor (grounding). She then translated Dani's emotion into words.

Marcia: "I see you are disappointed and even a bit angry."
Dani: "Yeaaah! I WANT THAT TOY!"
Marcia: "You really want that toy, and it makes you upset that you can't have it."
Dani: "Yeaaaah!"

Dani continued crying and yelling. Marcia held Dani and took him to a different part of the store, while trying to take long exhales to activate the parasympathetic nervous system to keep calm and so that Dani could 'borrow' some of that calmness.

What Dani learnt from this experience was

- To express anger in words (thus reducing the likelihood of using aggressive behaviours in expressing anger).
- To use a set of anger management skills (breathing, stepping away from the situation, calm down time).
- His mum will stay with him even when he is experiencing difficult times.
- Emotions are manageable and not a cause for disconnection from his parent.

You can use the following worksheet as a guide to have conversations with your child about emotions and self-management.

Worksheet 5.3 Anger management for children (Therapist Aid, n.d.)

Anger starts out small. This is when you start to feel upset about something. Sometimes people say they are 'annoyed' when they are feeling like this.

Draw what you look like when your anger is **small**. This is when you are just a little bit angry or annoyed.

| |
| |
| |

If your anger has the chance to grow too big, it can become harder to control. It is like a car without brakes, crashing through everything in its way. Someone who is this angry might shout, cry, hit others or break things. Draw what anger could look like when it is big.

Draw what it is like when your anger is **very big**.

| |
| |
| |

Worksheet 5.4 Anger stop signs (Therapist Aid, n.d.)

Anger stops signs are clues and signs our body uses to let us know our anger is growing big. The body starts sending us these signs when the anger is small, and as it gets bigger the signs get 'louder'. When we notice these signs we can pause and manage our anger in a way that won't hurt us or others.

Everyone has their own stop signs. It is important to know what yours are. Write/draw your anger stop sings below.

```
┌─────────────────────────────────────────┐
│                                         │
│                                         │
│                                         │
│                                         │
│                                         │
│                                         │
│                                         │
│                                         │
└─────────────────────────────────────────┘
```

Common anger stop signs:
My face feels hot.
I go quiet.
I can't think straight.
I can feel my heart beat faster.
I grind my teeth.
I start to shake.
I can't stay still.
My eyes get watery.
I raise my voice.
My leg muscles get tight.
I make a fist.
I want to hit something/someone.
My mouth becomes dry.

Sexual intelligence skills

Worksheet 5.5 What to do with my anger

All feelings are okay, but not all behaviours are okay. It is okay to feel VERY angry, but it is never okay to hit someone. We can do things to help us stay with the anger until it passes and listen to it to find out what it is trying to tell us.

Write down or draw some things you can do when you feel angry.

Some ideas: walk away (go to another room), talk to an adult or trusted person, push a wall, punch a pillow, run around the backyard, stomp your feet, take five deep breaths, put your headphones on and listen to loud music, jump on a trampoline, draw your anger.

Think about the last time you got angry. What do you think your anger was trying to tell you?

Some examples: When my sister broke my favourite toy my anger was telling me how much I loved that toy.

When other kids didn't let me play with them my anger was telling me I feel lonely if no one plays with me.

How do all of these relate to sexuality education, you may ask? Emotional intelligence means not only do we become more aware of our own emotions and can manage them, but also, we can become more aware of the other's internal state and respond accordingly.

Lack of empathy and a low level of emotional intelligence is at the core of sexual violence, assault and unhappy and unfulfilling sexual and romantic relationships. In relationships, low levels of empathy and emotional intelligence can lead to unhealthy power dynamics and lack of understanding. Partners may not be able to communicate their needs effectively, leading to feelings of frustration and resentment. This can create a toxic environment where one partner may feel pressured into engaging in sexual activities they are uncomfortable with or where emotional manipulation and abuse is present.

It is crucial to teach young people about empathy and emotional intelligence, as they are key components of healthy relationships and consensual sexual experiences. This includes understanding the importance of respecting boundaries, communicating openly and honestly, and recognising and managing emotions.

Luckily, empathy is a skill that can be taught and developed.

COMMUNICATION SKILLS

Empathy
Empathy is the ability to recognise the perspective of another person and to use that understanding to guide our actions. Empathy is not just a 'moral thing' to do or to have. Research shows that empathy increases the quality of our life and relationships (Rosenberg, 2018).

When you look at the definition of empathy you will see it doesn't say anything about agreeing with the other person's values or beliefs. Empathy is trying to understand a situation from another person's perspective.

However, recent research has shown that empathy also has a physiological basis. This is because when we closely observe another person's facial expressions, gestures and tone of voice, a process known as neural resonance occurs in our brains. Neural resonance is when our brain aligns with the other person's, allowing us to more accurately understand their emotions and experiences (Schaefer et al., 2012).

Researchers at Princeton University conducted an fMRI brain scan on participants and discovered that neural resonance disappeared when people communicated poorly (Stephens et al., 2010). Interestingly, the researchers could predict how well people were communicating by observing how much their brains were aligned. They found that people who were paying close attention could actually anticipate what the other person was about to say before they said it!

In this part I will share with you some practical skills that I learnt as a psychotherapist which helped me tap into my inner empathy more and be more in tune with other people.

Active listening skills

What successful hostage negotiators and psychotherapists know is that the key element in effective communication is *listening*.

Most often people *think* they are listening, but what they are doing is preparing what to say next when the other person stops talking. Active listening skills are rooted in curiosity to truly understand the other person's perspective. Listening seems like a passive activity, but it is in fact an active process and more difficult than it seems. We can get caught in our emotions, feel defensive and feel the urge to interrupt. We tend to engage in selective listening, hearing only what we want to hear, which means we will miss out on information which can help us solve the problem and move forward.

Psychology research shows that when someone feels listened to, they are more likely to evaluate and clarify their own emotions and consider the possible options (Fischer-Lokou et al., 2016). In addition, they tend to become less defensive and oppositional and more willing to listen to the other person's point of view. Don't we all love to talk to someone who is open to hearing our point of view?

In one of the most well-known research projects, George A. Miller (1956) concludes that humans can process only about seven pieces of information at any given time. For those people who tend to see communication and negotiation as an opportunity to prove their argument, it is the voice in their own head that is overwhelming them with more than seven pieces of information. When they are not talking, they are making their arguments and when they are talking, they are making their argument! Often both sides of the table are doing the same thing, so you have two people plus the voices in their head, that is over four people talking at the same time!

There is one powerful way to address this issue. Instead of doing any thinking about what you are going to say, make it your sole focus to understand the other person's perspective. In that state of trust and active listening (aided by some other tools which I will share with you) you will have a much higher chance of calming your mind, making rational decisions, as well as making the other person feel safe and therefore more open to what we have to say. If individuals feel safe and have a positive mindset, they are more likely to cooperate and work together to solve problems rather than confront and oppose the other person.

The first step in active listening is to become aware of your emotions and thoughts. So, the more aware we are of our internal thoughts and emotions the more likely it is to hold them and make a value-based decision rather than reacting to the situation.

Here is a technique I learnt as a psychotherapist which I use in all my interactions in life and have found it to work like a magic wand!

What is the message behind the words?

As a therapist it is important that you understand what the underlying emotions and thoughts of a person are which may be inhibiting their growth, as a result I have learnt to stay continuously curious about the other person's internal experiences and drives.

The capacity to reflect someone's internal state and without judgement is at the heart of all healthy relationships (romantic or otherwise). It also has a tremendous effect on calming the brain in the moment, meaning it will be easier to comfort someone as well as set boundaries and move to a productive and helpful place. When we reflect a person's inner thoughts and feelings with sincerity and curiosity, it activates a series of brain-based events that decreases the intensity of their emotional experience, even if you don't agree with them. It is a neurobiological response that involves different chemicals and parts of the brain that work together to send a signal to the brain: "I have been heard. I can calm down" (Phelan, 2020).

When a client (or a friend) tells me something, I try to understand what the message (emotions and thoughts) behind their words is. For example, one of my clients, let's call her Rosie, who was a single mother of a six-month-old baby and was homeless told me: "Do you have kids? Do you know how hard it is to live like this?" If we look at the surface of these questions we may respond: "Yes, I do have kids. I can imagine how hard it is for you." To which the client can respond: "No you can't! You have never slept rough with a hungry baby in your arms. You will never understand." And we would get in the vicious cycle of me wanting to prove to her that I can try to understand and she wanting to prove to me that it is impossible. However, when I identified the underlying feelings, I responded: "It sounds like you are worried I may not get what you are going through." To which she responded: "That's right." And when you get "That's right" from someone, there is a lot more opportunity for rapport and for moving towards a direction which is mutually beneficial.

Another client once told me: "Women are all manipulative and untrustworthy." My initial internal response was: "Well, not all women are like that." But then I realised that I was having an emotional reaction and I became aware of it. Then I asked myself: "What is he trying to say? What is the message behind the words?" After a moment I said: "It sounds like you have not been able to trust most women in your life." His response? "That's exactly RIGHT!"

What I love about this method is that you do not have to agree or disagree with the statement the other person is making. You do not have to answer a question just because it has been asked. You validate the person's emotions and experience, and BOOM trust and rapport is established or maintained.

So next time when someone says something to you, you can use the following starters to identify the emotions and thoughts behind the words and notice the effects:

"It sounds like. . . ."

"It seems like. . . ."

Or label the emotion: "You are worried that. . . ."

"You are frustrated because. . . ."

"You feel. . . ."

When we are able to reflect on the other person's emotional state and validate their experience and feelings (without necessarily agreeing with them) our chances of mutual respect, trust and connection increases exponentially. All of these qualities are fundamental in healthy, functioning sexual and romantic relationships (all relationships for that matter).

Being able to identify the other person's feelings and emotions take practice. You might get it wrong at first, but don't worry, the person will correct you and then you will know. I once told a client: "It sounds like you are frustrated with the situation." She said: "NO! I am fucking MAD!" *Oops! I got it wrong!* "So, you are infuriated!" to which she responded: "Exactly!"

Once you get the hang of this technique it will become your magic wand, valuable in every personal, professional and social setting. Use this with your children and see the calming effect it can have on them, making them more likely to listen to you, cooperate and even come up with their own solutions to problems!

How does this relate to sexuality education? Firstly, communication skills that people learn from other areas of life can be generalised to sexual situations. In addition, staying curious about the other person's emotions and internal state and the ability to listen actively to a partner is key in healthy relationships, sexual or otherwise. Finally, when communicating with your teen about topics which may be awkward or uncomfortable, this technique will help you navigate those challenges by identifying what your child may be experiencing. Here is an example:

Raya: Now that you and Peter are dating, I thought I would ask if you know where to get condoms from.
Jackson: MUM!!
Raya: You feel awkward about me bringing up this topic.
Jackson: Yes!
Raya: I know we haven't talked about this before, and we both may feel awkward, but I want you to know your health and safety matters to me. Let me know if you ever have questions or feel confused about things. Relationships can be confusing!
Jackson: Ok. Thanks.

And in a sexual relationship:

Rosie and Max have been together for three years. Rosie would like to have sex more often than does Max. This has created tension in the relationship and has affected other areas of their romantic relationship. Max tries to avoid any physical touch with the fear that Rosie may see this as an invitation to have intercourse. Rosie on the other hand feels frustrated that her needs are not being met in this relationship. She feels rejected and invalidated. She finally tells Max that if they don't address this issue she will have to leave.

How can Rosie and Max use the previous technique to communicate in a calm and productive manner about the issue and what is important for them?

Rosie: It looks like you avoid any physical touch and intimacy because you fear it may lead to intercourse and you are just not interested in intercourse as much as I am.

As you can see Rosie is just stating facts. She is not making any judgements or bringing her emotions or needs (yet) to the conversation.

Max: That's right.

How can Max reflect on Rosie's internal state?

Max: It seems like sexuality is an important part of the relationship for you. You feel rejected every time you initiate a physical touch and I refuse to engage.

Similarly, Max is reflecting on Rosie's internal state rather than finger pointing or telling her how *he* feels.

You may ask, but how can I communicate about my needs and expectations if the other person is not reflecting on my *internal* state?

This will take us to the next technique: intent-impact.

Intent-impact
Sometimes bringing up feelings to someone you care about can be nerve-racking. No one wants to feel like they're overreacting or causing a fuss. However, to maintain a healthy relationship with loved ones we need to be able to express how their behaviours impact us and what we expect from them.

Here is a typical scenario I hear in my therapy room, and I suspect it won't be unfamiliar to you:

Lola: I hate it when you creep up on me at night and grope me.
Matthew: I don't creep up on you. You are my wife! I want to make love to you. If I leave it up to you, it will never happen and then you complain about lack of intimacy. For God's sake, what do you want from me?

How could Lola express she is unhappy with the way her husband approaches her without hurting his feelings? We will come back to Lola and Matthew in a bit.

Before getting any further, it's important to understand how someone's intent differs from their impact. Intent is what they think or feel during an action or conversation. It's usually the reason or motivation behind the situation. Someone might explain their intent by saying, "Well, I said it that way because. . . ." or "what I meant was. . . ."

Impact refers to how that action or conversation makes the other person *feel*. They might bring up the issue of the impact by saying, "It made me feel. . . ."

In a nutshell, intent refers to what you were trying to do. Impact refers to how that action was perceived by the other person (Toscano, 2020).

Here are some examples of how intent and impact show up in everyday life:

- Your mother makes a joke that upsets you. You know that she didn't mean any harm, but it still stings. Her **intent** was light-hearted, but the **impact** is that your feelings are hurt.
- A friend comes to you to talk about an issue they're having with their partner. You offer them advice, but your friend is defensive and ends the conversation. You later learn that they felt like you were telling them they handled the situation poorly. Your **intent** was to help problem solve, but the **impact** was that they felt judged.
- Your employer introduces a new policy at work, but the staff feel like it's just more work and monitoring, exacerbating the lack of trust in the office. Your supervisor's **intent** was to add processes for efficiency, but the **impact** is a decrease in morale.
- Your teen brings home a report card that has grades lower than what's typical of them. You sit them down to have a

conversation about the importance of doing their best, and they shut down. It turns out they feel like your words are coming from a place of disappointment, not love or encouragement. Your **intent** was to foster a conversation about motivation, but the **impact** is that your teen felt judged.

If someone says you hurt them

If someone discloses that you hurt or offended them, this is how you can manage the situation (Toscano, 2020):

- Listen with the goal of understanding where they're coming from, not with the goal of defending yourself. It can help to use the active listening techniques to ensure they feel heard.
- Centre their feelings, not yours. It's normal to feel a little prickly when someone tells you that you did something wrong and you disagree. You can say something like: "It sounds like my joke made you feel hurt, although my intention was light-hearted."
- Genuinely apologise or acknowledge the impact that your actions had on them. Steer clear of "I'm sorry if", "I'm sorry that you feel" or "I'm sorry but", as these all lack accountability and put the blame on the one who was hurt. A simple "I'm sorry for doing that" can go a long way.
- Ask them how they would like you to do it differently next time. If you are unclear about what is expected of you or what caused the hurt then it is difficult if not impossible not to repeat it.

If you want to talk to someone about how they made you feel (Toscano, 2020)

- Get curious about their intent. Why do you think they did that? Most often the intent is not causing you harm. For example: "I think your intent was to remind me of my responsibilities at home" or "I think your intent was to express your frustration with the situation."
- Focus on your feelings (the impact) and use 'I' statements. For example, you could say "I felt really hurt when. . . ."

instead of "You hurt me when. . . ." This centres the conversation on the impact the action had on you versus the situation itself or placing blame on the other person. Or you could say something like: "I think your intent is to protect our kids and to show how much you love them, but the impact of the way you said it is that I felt really hurt."
- Discuss how the situation could have been handled differently. Is there anything the other person could do differently if this situation happens again?

Now let's go back to Lola and Mathew. This is how Lola could express her feelings using this technique:

Lola: I know when you approach me at night and touch me, you want to show that you desire me and want to have sex, but it makes me feel unsafe. Can you instead tell me verbally when you want to initiate sex?

Mirroring

Mirroring is another technique psychotherapists use to establish trust and facilitate communication. Mirroring (its fancy term is isopraxim) is a non-verbal neurobehavior in which members of a species act in a similar manner. This means we copy each other's behaviour non-consciously to create safety and to comfort each other. It creates a sense of safety and comfort, indicating that people are bonding and establishing rapport. It is done with speech patterns, body language, vocabulary, tempo and tone of voice. Although it is a non-conscious behaviour, we can practise it to utilise it consciously and effectively.

Mirroring also helps to facilitate empathy, as we more readily experience other people's emotions through mimicking their posture and gestures. So, if you want to understand the other person's emotions better, literally hold their body posture, their tone of voice and their gestures.

If you pay attention to the environment you will notice mirroring everywhere: couples walking with their steps in perfect sync, in a group of people you may notice individuals adopting similar postures or gestures. Parents and caregivers also use mirroring when they interact with babies and young children. They often mirror the child's facial expressions, cooing sounds and body movements to establish a connection and create a sense of safety and comfort.

Psychologist Richard Wiseman conducted a study to determine the most effective way to establish a connection with someone you don't know. He asked a group of waiters to either repeat the customer's order or use positive reinforcement, such as "great!", "no problem" and "of course". The waiters who repeated the customer's order received a 70% higher tip on average than those who used positive reinforcement (Voss & Raz, 2016).

Many people think mirroring would feel awkward or that the other person would notice it and get offended. Speaking from experience I can tell you it will feel awkward the first few times you use it. Listening skills like any other skills become easier and a second nature the more you practise them. As for the other person finding out, it is very unlikely. As long as you do give a few seconds before mimicking their body language and posture, they will not notice it. As I said, it is a natural part of being a human, so we are used to others attuning to us and mirroring our behaviours. Even if they do find out you are doing something unusual you can be transparent and tell them about the new technique you have learnt to understand their point of view better. I can't imagine someone arguing with that point!

So, what does this look like in the context of sexuality education? Firstly, these skills will come to your aid when you want to talk to your child about sexuality. By identifying the emotions and thoughts driving their behaviour, you are more likely able to provide them with the information that is useful to them rather than random facts and figures. Empathy and communication skills can help you both (or all) move from a point of pressure towards problem solving together. One of my clients, Susi, after learning about communication skills, decided to implement them in her interactions and communications with her 17-year-old son.

Felix came home one day after his curfew time. I was worried sick and as soon as he entered the house I wanted to blow-up! I realised I was super angry. I took a long breath and labelled my emotion. *I am feeling angry.* While I was reflecting on my feelings, Felix said: "Mum I am sorry I'm late. I was dropping off Natasha. She didn't have a ride." My first reaction was *you could have bloody phoned me!* Then I tried to put myself in his shoes. He was trying to help a friend, and I had taught him myself to drop people off if they needed a ride and not to leave them stranded. So I said: "You wanted to make sure Natasha got home safe." He looked at me and said: "That's right. I know it's late, and you were probably expecting a call from me, but my phone's battery died." I couldn't help but let the drama queen inside me to rush to him and give him a big hug! I am so glad I didn't blow up like I would most of the time, otherwise it would have ended in me shouting at him even before giving him a chance to explain why he was late, by which time it was too late, I would have hurt him and felt guilt and self-hatred for the rest of the week.

By practising these communication skills and incorporating them into your everyday life you will be providing your young person with the opportunity to learn some very effective skills for their current and future relationships, including romantic and sexual relationships. Attunement and empathy combined with sound communication skills are a guaranteed recipe for healthy and functional relationships.

Dr Rebecca Ray, in her book *Setting Boundaries*, introduces the acronym LISTEN to remember the fundamentals of active listening skills (Ray, 2021):

Lean in and pay attention

Impartial attitude

Share what you're hearing

Test understanding

Encouragers

No-pressure summary

Lean in and pay attention
Lean in slightly towards the other person and give them your full attention. Our body posture and non-verbal language communicates a lot more than our words.

Impartial attitude
Even if the person is saying something that you don't like, as much as possible try to remain open-minded and non-judgemental. This helps hearing their perspective with as little interpretation (we can never completely remove it) from our side. (For example: "I feel I don't have enough space in this relationship" doesn't necessarily mean "I want to end the relationship.")

Share what you're hearing
Reflect back what you're hearing by paraphrasing after each significant point made by the other person. You can use the following starters to paraphrase what you have heard:

- What I'm hearing is. . . .
- Sounds like you are saying. . . .
- If I'm hearing you correctly. . . .
- So, as you see it. . . .
- It sounds like what's most important to you is. . . .

For example: "I couldn't sleep last night because I was angry you were making so much noise. I had to take care of the kids as well as prepare for tomorrow's presentation! How can you be so selfish?"

Paraphrase: "Sounds like you got really stressed out and angry last night because of all the noise I made. You had to take care of the kids on top of preparing for your work presentation."

Test understanding
Ask questions to clarify anything you are unclear about.

Example: "Let me see if I understand you correctly. You admire my commitment to work, but when I am late it makes you feel like I am not committed to our family. Is that right?"

Or

"Wait, I am not sure I am following you. Could you be more specific? What do you mean by...?"

Or

"Can you explain that to me a little bit more?"

Encouragers
Encouragers are words or noises like 'Mmm hmm', 'I see', 'go on' and/or non-verbal minimal encouragers such as eye contact, head nods and smiles. We use encouragers to:

- Show we are tracking the conversation
- Remain neutral

No-pressure summary
Summarise the important parts of the conversation and how the person is feeling. You don't have to get it perfectly right and repeat everything. If you have misunderstood something the person will correct you. As long as the other person feels heard and sees your effort to understand them, you are on the way to a meaningful and productive communication.

Tips for active listening (Ray, 2021)
- Listen more than you speak. Aim to do 80% listening and 20% talking to give the other person space to deliver their message.
- Listen to what is being said rather than plan for what you want to say next.

- Avoid interrupting the speaker.
- Avoid jumping in with advice giving or problem solving unless it is asked for. Most often all people need is to feel heard.
- Move away from distractions. Devices, TV, kids, etc. can impair everyone's ability to concentrate.
- Avoid speaking to fill silence. Silence can be a powerful tool. It allows both parties to collect their thoughts, reflect on what was said, consider how they want to proceed and process their feelings.
- Avoid telling the other person they shouldn't be *feeling* the way they feel. Telling someone they shouldn't feel the way they do invalidates their experience. Acknowledging their feelings doesn't mean you agree with their point of view.

CRITICAL THINKING SKILLS

There are times in everyone's life that they may not want to or have the opportunity to share things with their parents. As difficult as it is for us as parents to accept this, we need to respect this right. However, we need to make sure our children know how to make sound decisions for themselves. Sometimes unexpected things happen, maybe your family goes through a rough time, maybe you are not physically available to your child for a variety of legitimate reasons, but by guiding and teaching your child to seek information from trusted sources you are teaching them a life skill that can help them in many aspects of their lives, including their sexuality. The reality is we will not be there with them during every moment of their lives. Moreover, in the Information Age, where research data and information are updated every second, we cannot possibly teach them all they need to know! So instead of giving them a fish let's teach them how to fish.

We make hundreds if not thousands of decisions every day, although we may not be aware of them. Choosing to sleep in five more minutes or to get up, what clothes to wear, whether to check social media the first thing in the morning, what to eat, how to respond to our partner, children, colleagues, the list is endless. Some decisions have a much more significant impact than others, for example, whether to go on a date with someone we fancy or the career path we choose.

Critical thinking skills can help us make decisions which are less reactive and more logical and well-informed. Critical thinking is the analysis of a question or situation and the facts, data or evidence related to it. When we consider a question/argument critically we become aware of our own emotions, opinions and biases and those of the others involved, and we look at it from different perspectives.

Most often when we are presented with information it is one-sided, meaning some other point or views are missing. For example, I just typed in Google 'drinking coffee' and clicked on the first article suggested: '9 Reasons Why (the Right Amount of) Coffee Is Good for You'. Here are the main points from this article:

> You could live longer.
>
> Your body may process glucose (or sugar) better.
>
> You're less likely to develop heart failure.
>
> You are less likely to develop Parkinson's disease.
>
> Your liver will thank you.
>
> Your DNA may be stronger.
>
> Your odds of getting colon cancer will go way down.
>
> You may decrease your risk of getting Alzheimer's disease.
>
> You're not as likely to suffer a stroke.

Sounds wonderful! It makes you want to drink coffee 25 times a day! But there are many points here which don't make this article a reliable and 'objective' source of information to make a decision about whether I should consider increasing my coffee intake. Let's go through them one by one:

- Firstly, and obviously, the opposing view (the reasons not to drink coffee) is missing, so it is one-sided, which doesn't discredit the source of information entirely, but it means before making a decision I should consider the other point(s) of view as well. So, a question I always ask when evaluating a piece of information or situation is "whose voice/view is missing?" It doesn't mean the other view is right, but it means I will have a broader source to guide my decision.
- Secondly, I have questions about the sources of the claims. There are several references to research without citing the research. This reduces the credibility of the source significantly. When looking for information about sex and sexuality encourage your child to question the credibility of the source of information (as a rule of thumb information in published books, journal articles, statistics and data on government websites, university websites, known health clinics, etc. are more reliable than random forums or social media).
- Third, there are very general claims without substantial back-ups. For example, "You could live longer." What does this mean? Everyone *could*! Longer compared to whom? By what percent? Is it a meaningful comparison and conclusion? For example, if one research shows people who drink coffee are 0.0000004% more likely to live one day longer than others, would that be a meaningful reason to drink coffee?
- Looking at the language, we can see a lot of 'mays' and 'mights', which don't make for a solid argument. "You may decrease your risk of getting Alzheimer's disease" or "Your DNA may be stronger."

There are a few principles that can guide critical thinking skills:

1. Objectivity: Critical thinking requires an objective approach that is free from personal biases, prejudices or emotional reactions.

Questions to ask:

- Am I basing my decisions on facts and evidence or on personal opinions and biases?
- Whose voice/point of view is missing here?
- Am I being fair and impartial in my evaluation?

2. Clarity: Critical thinking involves the ability to clearly articulate and express ideas and concepts, as well as to understand them when presented by others.

Questions to ask:

- Can I explain my decision clearly and concisely to others?
- Have I identified and defined all the key terms and concepts involved in the decision?
- Am I using language that is precise and easily understandable?

3. Open-mindedness: Critical thinking involves being open to new ideas and perspectives and being willing to consider evidence that challenges one's beliefs and assumptions.

Questions to ask:

- Am I willing to consider alternative viewpoints and ideas?
- Am I willing to challenge my own assumptions and biases?

4. Curiosity: Critical thinking requires a curious mind that seeks to understand, explore and ask questions about the world.

Questions to ask:

- Am I asking questions and seeking to understand the issue more deeply?
- Am I exploring different perspectives and seeking out new information?
- Am I willing to learn from others and consider their viewpoints?

5. Metacognition: Critical thinking involves being aware of one's own thought processes and biases and being able to reflect on and evaluate one's own thinking.

Questions to ask:

- Am I aware of my own biases and assumptions?
- Have I evaluated my own thought processes and decision-making strategies?
- Am I willing to reflect on my decisions and learn from my mistakes?

6. Research: When comparing points of view and making important decisions, independent research ability is key. Arguments are *meant* to be persuasive. That means the facts and figures presented in their favour might be lacking the context or come from questionable sources or be presented in misleading ways. The best way to counter this is independent evaluation. Find the source of the information and evaluate.

Questions to ask:

- Does the person posing the argument offer where they got this information from?
- If you ask or try to find it yourself is there a clear answer?

7. Identify biases: Even empirical research can be biased and lack objectivity. Sometimes, the funder of a research paper or study has a vested interest in the research 'proving' a certain point. For example, while studying for my bachelor's degree, I once came across a research project that explored the effects of tobacco and alcohol on driving. The results showed that people who drank alcohol and smoked before driving had a very marginal decrease in reaction time compared to those who only drank alcohol. The researchers then concluded that smoking tobacco after drinking alcohol can reduce reaction time and decrease the risk of collisions! It would not be surprising to learn that the funder of the research was a tobacco company. Unfortunately, I could not find the research to cite it.

Questions to ask:

- Who does this benefit?
- Does the source of this information appear to have an agenda?
- Is the source overlooking, ignoring or leaving out information that doesn't support its beliefs or claims?

- Is this source using unnecessary language to sway an audience's perception of a fact?
- What other information would make me reconsider this decision/conclusion?

8. Curiosity: Critical thinking requires a curious mind that seeks to understand, explore and ask questions about the world.

Questions to consider:

- How do I know this?
- Who taught me that?
- Where do I get this idea from?
- What happens if I assume the exact opposite?
- Am I holding this belief because everyone else around me is?

Teaching our children the skills for critical thinking and the ability to objectively analyse and evaluate complex subjects and situations can help them make informed decisions in their life. Important decisions such as the time and situation in which they engage in sexual activities, the partners they choose, the type of sexual activities, conforming or opposing societal norms and many many more significant choices they make.

REFERENCE LIST

Cotruş, A., Stanciu, C., & Bulborea, A. (2012). EQ vs. IQ which is most important in the success or failure of a student? *Procedia, Social and Behavioral Sciences, 46*, 5211–5213. https://doi.org/10.1016/j.sbspro.2012.06.411

Curtis, E. (2021, January 18). 6 Things emotionally intelligent parents do differently. *Psychology Today.* https://www.psychologytoday.com/au/blog/the-therapist-mommy/202101/6-things-emotionally-intelligent-parents-do-differently

Fischer-Lokou, J., Lamy, L., Guéguen, N., & Dubarry, A. (2016). Effects of active listening, reformulation, and imitation on mediator success: Preliminary results. *Psychological Reports, 118*(3), 994–1010. https://doi.org/10.1177/0033294116646159

Gottman, J. (2018). Emotional intelligence creates loving and supportive parenting. *The Gottman Institute.* Retrieved May 28, 2021, from https://www.gottman.com/blog/emotional-intelligence-creates-loving-supportive-parenting/

Heydari, M., Masafi, S., Jafari, M., Saadat, S., & Shahyad, S. (2018). Effectiveness of acceptance and commitment therapy on anxiety and depression of Razi Psychiatric Center staff. *Open Access Macedonian Journal of Medical Sciences, 6*(2), 410–415. https://doi.org/10.3889/oamjms.2018.064

La Trobe University. (2021). Why emotional intelligence makes you more successful. *Nest*. Retrieved May 28, 2021, from https://www.latrobe.edu.au/nest/why-emotional-intelligence-makes-you-more-successful/#:~:text=Emotional%20intelligence%20is%20the%20ability,conflict%20and%20improve%20job%20satisfaction.&text=EI%20is%20important%20for%20everyone%20who%20wants%20to%20be%20career%20ready

Mahtani, A. (2020). Square breathing technique: How-to and benefits. *Medical News Today*.

Matthews, G., Deary, I. J., & Whiteman, M. C. (2012). *Personality traits* (3rd ed.). Cambridge University Press.

Mayer, J. D., Salovey, P., & Caruso, D. R. (2004). Emotional intelligence: Theory, findings, and implications. *Psychological Inquiry, 15*(3), 197–215.

Miller, G. (1956). The magical number seven, plus or minus two: Some limits on our capacity for processing information. *Psychological Review, 63*(2), 81–97. https://doi.org/10.1037/h0043158

Phelan, T. W. (2020). *What to say to kids when nothing seems to work*. Sourcebooks.

Ray, R. (2021). *Setting boundaries*. Pan Macmillan Australia.

Rosenberg, M. (2018). Empathy and quality of life. In S. K. Bardzil & M. A. Jenkins (Eds.), *The handbook of empathy* (pp. 401–413). Routledge.

Schaefer, M., Heinze, H., & Rotte, M. (2012). Embodied empathy for tactile events: Interindividual differences and vicarious somatosensory responses during touch observation. *NeuroImage, 60*(2), 952–957. https://doi.org/10.1016/j.neuroimage.2012.01.112

Stephens, G., Silbert, L., & Hasson, U. (2010). Speaker–listener neural coupling underlies successful communication. *Proceedings of the National Academy of Sciences—PNAS, 107*(32), 14425–14430. https://doi.org/10.1073/pnas.1008662107

Therapist Aid. (n.d.). Anger warning signs for children. https://www.therapistaid.com/worksheets/anger-warning-signs-children

Torre, J., & Lieberman, M. (2018). Putting feelings into words: Affect labeling as implicit emotion regulation. *Emotion Review, 10*(2), 116–124. https://doi.org/10.1177/1754073917742706

Toscano, J. (2020, June 22). Intent vs. impact: What's the difference and why does it matter? *Healthline*. https://www.healthline.com/health/intent-vs-impact#the-difference

Voss, C., & Raz, T. (2016). *Never split the difference: Negotiating as if your life depended on it* (1st ed.). HarperBusiness, an Imprint of HarperCollins Publishers.

Watkins, D., & Huang, L. (2003). The efficacy of mindfulness-based interventions in reducing symptoms of depression: A meta-analysis. *Journal of Counseling Psychology, 50*(2), 279–283. https://doi.org/10.1037/0022-0167.50.2.279

CHAPTER 6

A strength-based approach

When Janet asked her 17-year-old son, Kyle, if he uses condoms when he has sex, Kyle's response was: "yeah, half of the time." Janet felt disheartened that all her efforts throughout the years teaching her son about STIs and the risk of unintended pregnancy was futile. *You're only using condoms half of the time?! That's a pretty big risk to take. You could get STIs, including HIV, and you could get someone pregnant*, was what she wanted to shout out loud! After taking a breath and becoming aware of her emotions, she remembered her core values of respect and love and decided to respond in a different way: "That's great that you're using condoms! I'm curious, what's been working for you during the times when you do use them?" Kyle disclosed to his mum that he would use them when he knew there was a chance to have sex with his girlfriend and the times things happened spontaneously, he just let it go. They were then able to brainstorm about how he could have more frequent access to condoms. Janet also referred him to a website with information on lower-risk sexual activities, such as oral sex, mutual masturbation and erotic massage.

Using a strength-based approach we acknowledge that the young person, when given access to accurate age-appropriate information, has the capacity to make good decisions for their life. It means listening to our children with respect and trying to understand their point of view. When we approach the matter with curiosity and respect we can often find solutions to barriers young people face.

Strength-based approach:

- Approaching the matter with curiosity.
- Providing accurate information.

DOI: 10.4324/9781003435600-9

- Expressing empathy.
- Encouraging the young person to see the problem from the point of view of the other person/people involved.

Let's have a look at a scenario and see what a strength-based approach can look like in practice:

> Selma is 15 years old and has been in a relationship with Lola, a 16-year-old girl, for three weeks. Selma's father, Alex, notices that she seems excited and energetic every day when she wakes up. She spends over three hours on the phone with Lola every day and is considering announcing their relationship at her upcoming birthday party next week. Alex is concerned that Selma is rushing things and is worried about the impact of the relationship on Selma's education and schooling. Alex decides to talk to Selma about his concerns.
>
> When Selma enters the kitchen to make a snack, Alex says, "Selma, don't you think you're rushing things with Lola? I haven't even met her yet, and you're already planning to announce your relationship next week. You've been with her for less than a month! I'm also concerned that all the time you're spending on the phone with her is taking you away from your studies."

What do you think Alex's intention behind this statement is? What do you think the potential impact could be on Selma?

Selma feels furious that her dad doesn't get her.

> "How can you doubt my decision? She is the best thing that has ever happened me! I was planning to bring her home tomorrow to meet you! Besides, I am in a much better mood thanks to her, so it means I can do my homework much faster than I used to. But you don't get it, do you?"
>
> "I would love to meet her, but I am thinking you are taking it too fast. I don't want you to feel heartbroken again."
>
> "You don't even know her. How can you judge?" Selma stomps out of the room.

A strength-based approach

Now, let's see how this could look with a strength-based approach. This is obviously one potential way the conversation could go, but I hope it can help you see what it can look like when applied in everyday interactions.

When Selma enters the kitchen to make herself a snack, Alex says, "You look like you're in an exceptionally good mood these days. I'd love to hear more about what's going on for you and how your relationship with Lola is going."

Selma grins and says, "Dad, you have no idea. She is the best thing that has ever happened to me. It sounds like she can hear my thoughts before I even think them!"

"Sounds like you feel connected with her."

"That's right! I just can't wait to let everyone know we are in a relationship. She is so beautiful and smart and cool!"

"I would love to meet her! Can we make some time in the next couple of days for me to meet her?"

"Yeah, we were thinking tomorrow."

"Awesome! Can't wait. I'd love to hear more about what's happening for you and your relationship with Lola."

"Maybe tonight when you pick me up from ballet?"

"Great."

Six hours later in the car.

"I'm really pleased to see you excited and full of energy all the time, Selma. It reminds me of when I was in love for the first time."

"Was it mum?"

"No, it was a girl from high school. Vanessa. We used to talk on the landline the whole time. I remember the feeling. I had butterflies in my stomach all the time. You spend quite a lot of time on the phone with Lola too, don't you?"

"I know. We just can't get enough of each other."

"I can imagine. I am a little worried about the effect on your schooling, though. What are your thoughts on that?"

Selma grunts.

"I know you're 15 and you want to make decisions for your life and relationship. I am worried, though, that suddenly having three hours less in a day can impact your grades. You studied really hard this year, and I would hate to see you not getting the grades you wanted."

Selma doesn't say anything.

Alex is silent for a minute. "You are quiet. Is it because you are disappointed? Is there maybe something there that I am not seeing?"

"No. Yes, I am disappointed because I don't want to think about school. I know I need to spend more time studying, but it's hard because I would like to spend every waking moment with my girlfriend! Life SUCKS!"

"I hear you are conflicted."

"Yeah. I don't know. I'll think about it. It's hard, Dad, you know?"

"I know, sweetie. Having a relationship and other responsibilities in life is not an easy task."

"Are you implying Lola and I will not be together forever?"

"I don't know. You may or you may not. What I am saying is you are becoming an adult, and this is one part of being an adult. If you ever have any questions or are confused about anything, you know you can talk to me or mum, right?"

"Yeah, I know."

"So, what time am I seeing Lola tomorrow? How do you want me to dress for the occasion?"

CHAPTER 7
Value-based decision-making

> The secret of man's being is not only to live, but to have something to live for.
>
> (Fyodor Dostoyevsky)

Values are the fundamental beliefs we hold about how we should live, and they play a crucial role in determining our priorities. Values are measures we use to gauge if our life is moving in the direction we desire. When our actions and behaviours align with our values, we tend to feel content and satisfied. However, when we act in ways that are inconsistent with our values, we experience a sense of dissatisfaction and unhappiness. Whether or not we are aware of them, our values shape our lives, and acknowledging them can lead to a more fulfilling existence. By making choices and plans that are consistent with our values, we can create a more meaningful and satisfying life.

Research on acceptance and commitment therapy, motivational interviewing, and mindfulness-based approaches shows when people have a clear set of core values (Mikulak, 2016):

- It's easier to make big life decisions around pursuing long-term goals, careers and relationships.
- They are less likely to engage in destructive thought patterns, especially in difficult life situations.
- They have greater self-discipline and focus.
- Their social connections are stronger.

Teaching our kids to make value-based decisions can lead them to making better decisions that are fulfilling to them.

This includes decisions in the realm of relationships and sexuality. It can help them answer questions like these:

What kind of relationship do I want?

Should I compromise or be firm with my criteria for a relationship?

What kind of sexual encounters do I really want?

What kind of things am I willing to sacrifice in order to have that kind of relationship?

What do I value in a partner?

What do I value in being single?

Imagine this scenario: Jack values family and a stable romantic and sexual relationship but is pressured by his peers to have sex with a different girl every weekend. Would he feel internal stress and conflict? I would say so.

Natasha values spontaneity and health. When her boyfriend of two weeks asks her to have intercourse, she would like to say yes in the moment. She has packed a couple of condoms in her bag in case she is in a situation where she wants to decide spontaneously. Would she feel conflicted by her values in this way? Probably not.

So, taking the time to understand what values are important to us and what the real priorities are in our life, we will be able to determine the best direction for our life and our life goals.

DEFINING YOUR VALUES

Let us begin by looking inward to discover what really matters to you. When you define your personal values, you discover what is truly important to you. A good way of starting to do this is to look back on your life—to identify when you felt fulfilled and really confident that you were making good choices.

Step 1: Identify the times when you were authentic
When you're in situations that allow you to be authentic, that's a sign that you are in alignment with your values. And when we behave in ways to only fit in or find success in ways that is defined by others, we most often feel unfulfilled, burnt out or chronically angry.

Worksheet 7.1 Identifying times when you were authentic

In situations that feel wrong in some way, what is going on? Write down:

- Who you're with

- What activities are involved

- What feelings you experience

- What these experiences cost you (emotionally, psychologically or even physically)

In situations where you feel real and authentic, what is going on? Write down:

- Who you're with

- What activities are involved

- What feelings you experience

- What you gain by these experiences (emotionally, psychologically or even physically)

Step 2: Identify your drives

Often our core values reveal themselves through our actions. Think of a situation when you took a stand for someone or something (including your children).

> **Worksheet 7.2   Identifying your drives**
>
> Try writing down some of the reasons you felt so strong about taking action. For example:
>
> - The feelings that motivated you to speak up or act
>
> - What you were willing to risk in that situation?
>
> - The consequences of taking action—what you gained or lost

Step 3: Identifying who you admire

To gain a deeper understanding of your values, it can be helpful to look to individuals who demonstrate qualities that you admire. Consider positive role models who motivate you to live a fulfilling life, whether they are acquaintances, well-known individuals, or fictional characters from movies or literature. As you think about these people, write down:

> **Worksheet 7.3   Identifying who you admire**
>
> - What specifically about them is inspiring to you
>
> - The admirable qualities they show
>
> - The actions and behaviours you would like to model after them

Sexual intelligence skills

Step 4: Determine your top values, based on your sense of fulfilment

> **Worksheet 7.4   Determining your top values**
>
> Use the following list of common personal values to help you get started—and aim for about ten top values. (As you work through, you may find that some of these naturally overlap. For instance, if you value philanthropy, community and generosity, you might say that service to others is one of your top values.)

Core values list

Family	Freedom	Security	Loyalty
Intelligence	Connection	Creativity	Humanity
Success	Respect	Invention	Diversity
Generosity	Integrity	Finesse	Love
Openness	Religion	Order	Advancement
Respect	Joy/Play	Forgiveness	Excitement
Change	Goodness	Involvement	Faith
Wisdom	Beauty	Care	
Personal development	Honesty	Adventure	Kindness
Teamwork	Career	Communication	Learning
Excellence	Innovation	Quality	Commonality
Contributing	Spiritualism	Strength	Entertain
Wealth	Speed	Power	Affection
Cooperation	Friendship	Relationship	Encouragement
Pride	Clarity	Enjoyment	Charisma
Humour	Leadership	Renewal	Home
Authenticity	Contentment	Courage	Balance
Compassion	Fitness	Professionalism	Knowledge
Patience	Change	Prosperity	Wellness
Finances	Gratitude	Grace	Endurance
Facilitation	Effectiveness	Fame	Justice
Appreciation	Willingness	Intuition	Forgiveness
Self-respect	Abundance	Reciprocity	Entrepreneurial
Happiness	Harmony	Peace	

Step 5: Prioritise your top values

This step is probably the most difficult because you'll have to look deep inside yourself. It's also the most important step, because, when making a decision, you'll have to choose between solutions that may satisfy different values or if they are both of the same importance, to come up with solutions that satisfy both and not just the one.

Worksheet 7.5   Prioritising your top values

Write down your top values, not in any particular order.

Look at the first two values and ask yourself, "If I could satisfy only one of these, which would I choose?" It might help to visualise a situation in which you would have to make that choice. For example, you may need to choose between "financial stability" and "spending quality time with family". If you were offered a job opportunity that required you to work long hours and weekends, but with a higher salary, you may have to choose between the financial stability the job provides and the time you would have to spend away from your family. In this scenario, you would need to consider which value is more important to you and choose accordingly.

Step 6: Revaluate your values

Check your top-priority values and make sure that they fit with your life and your vision for yourself.

Worksheet 7.6   Revaluating your values

Do these values make you feel good about yourself?

Do these values represent things that are deep down important to you even if your choice isn't popular and it puts you in the minority?

When you consider your values in decision-making, you can be sure to keep your sense of integrity and what feels right, and you can approach decisions with confidence and clarity. You will also know that what you're doing is best for your current and future happiness and satisfaction.

Making value-based choices may not always be easy. However, making a choice that feels right is a lot less difficult and much more satisfying in the long run. Value-based decision-making can help our children to come up with ways to deal with unwanted sexual pressure, including peer pressure, and to make decisions that are more fulfilling for them in the long run. Let's keep in mind that we all make mistakes and make wrong decisions, including our children. Making mistakes is part of the journey of growth. If throughout the previous activities you realised you have made decisions that do not algin with your core values, be gentle with yourself. Refer to your self-compassion strategies and think about how you would like to incorporate value-based decision-making in your life and how to role model that for your children.

QUESTIONS FOR VALUE-BASED DECISION-MAKING

When you are faced with a difficult decision, consider using the following questions to make a value-based decision:

1. What decision are you considering? What are your options?
2. How do your options algin with your values?
3. How do your options conflict with your values?
4. Which values do you have to absolutely honour?
5. Which values are you willing to compromise?
6. Based on your previous answers, which decision is the best fit for your values? Why?

You can teach children about values directly and indirectly. One way to incorporate values education into our parenting is to express values in our communication with children. For example, if we want our five-year-old to help clean up after dinner we can say: "We **respect** each other by cleaning up after ourselves." Or to remind our 11-year-old about walking the family dog, we can say: "We all **contribute** to taking care of our pets because we are all **responsible** for our pets' wellbeing" (Center for Parenting Education, n.d.).

It is easy to get hyper-focused on whose turn it is to feed the cats or wash the dishes. By bringing the discussion back to the guiding values those tasks represent (empathy, responsibility, kindness), we can help our kids build a strong foundation for making value-based decisions.

A young person faced with an opportunity to be unfaithful to their partner may think: "I don't want to get caught. My partner will leave me if he finds out." Or "Honesty is important to me. It just wouldn't feel right to cheat."

When parents emphasise values such as respect, responsibility, integrity and empathy it creates a guideline for every decision: "Is this consistent with what I value?"

Worksheet 7.7 Value-based communication

Take a few moments and consider what values underlie these statements and you can reframe them when communicating with your children. I have included some examples as well:

> Don't hit your sister!
>
> Don't leave your clothes on the floor!
>
> Put that phone down!
>
> Don't interrupt me!
>
> Don't lose your jacket again!

Examples:

Respect: "You are frustrated. I get that. Please use your words instead of hitting your sister."
Responsibility: "We all love a clean and tidy house, so please put your clothes in the hamper."
Consideration: "You seem distracted. This conversation is important for me. Can you please focus on what I am saying for a few minutes without any distractions?"
Respect: "I'm speaking right now, please wait until I am finished and you will have my full attention."
Accountability: "What can help you remember where you leave your jacket?"

I cannot emphasise enough the importance of modelling the behaviour we want to see in our children. If we expect them to put away their phone when we are talking, we need to model that behaviour first. If we want them to show respectful behaviour towards people of all genders, we need to demonstrate that in our interactions and communication with others. Children learn by observing much more than what they are taught verbally.

It is crucial to remember that values are dynamic, not static. Therefore, it is essential to review them periodically throughout your life. Values are subject to change based on our circumstances and needs. For example, as someone from a collective culture, when I relocated to Australia in my early twenties, I began to value individualism and personal space more than community. However, after having a child, my values shifted, and I now value community living and resource-sharing more. As values change over time, it is important to re-evaluate them regularly to ensure they serve us and bring fulfilment. It's essential to assess whether the values we learned growing up or acquired during our lives are still relevant or not.

REFERENCE LIST

Center for Parenting Education. (n.d.). *Values-based parenting: Guideposts for choices.* https://centerforparentingeducation.org/library-of-articles/indulgence-values/values-based-parenting-guideposts-for-choices/

Mikulak, A. (2016). The heart of the matter. *Association for Psychological Science—APS.* Retrieved May 28, 2021, from https://www.psychologicalscience.org/observer/the-heart-of-the-matter

CHAPTER 8
Healthy boundaries

Setting healthy boundaries is one of the key elements of healthy sexual and romantic relationships. Healthy boundaries help us maintain a level of self-respect and communicate our wants and needs respectfully to our partner/s. Setting boundaries not only creates a safer space for sex and intimacy, but a more pleasurable one.

Unfortunately, many adults enter adulthood without having learnt the ability to recognise their own self-worth, trust their own judgement, and establish appropriate boundaries (Ray, 2021).

When Lukas sat down in my therapy room for the first time, he explained he was in a loving relationship with the woman of his dreams, but since dating her he had trouble getting an erection when having sex with her. "I don't understand. She is the sexiest and most wonderful woman I have ever met; I don't know why my body is behaving in this way!" After a few sessions, together we discovered that he always prioritised others' needs and pleasure over his. He had an open-door policy at work and in his personal life. He had been taking care of his ill father for over a decade and was emotionally burnt out. Lukas expressed he had this underlying 'guilt' all through his life and he tried to soothe the feeling by trying harder, but it felt as if he was never enough.

When discussing what he wanted for his life and from a relationship, Lukas had difficulty identifying anything other than "making others happy". This was Lukas's biggest gift and the underlying reason for the sexual challenges he was experiencing. He expressed that he didn't know what he wanted in a sexual relationship and in the instances that he knew what they were he was uncomfortable communicating them with his partner out of the fear that she would think he was not as good as her previous sexual partners, so he would focus on her pleasure and what she wanted.

Lukas was a caring and loving son and partner, but his lack of ability to set healthy boundaries with his loved ones was detrimental to his health and the quality of his relationship.

As you can see the concept of boundaries is closely intertwined with our sense of self-worth. Children who grow up to have a healthy sense of self experience more fulfilling relationships. But if we have never had the opportunity to learn about healthy boundaries, how can we teach and, more importantly, role model it? Next are the fundamentals of setting healthy boundaries. Most of this section comes from *Setting Boundaries* by Dr Rebecca Ray, as I found this book super helpful with lots of practical strategies to identify and set healthy boundaries. I highly recommend reading this book.

WHAT ARE BOUNDARIES?

Boundaries are like structures that safeguard our emotional and physical well-being. Without them, our emotional, psychological and physical resources are available to anyone, which can lead to chaos in our lives. Boundaries communicate to others the behaviours that we will and will not tolerate. Boundaries help to (Ray, 2021):

- Show others how to respect you. For example: dishonesty is a dealbreaker for many people.
- Distribute your personal resources effectively and accurately. For example: if I am taking care of three children full-time, can we come up with a plan to reduce my other chores at home?

- Demonstrate self-respect by defining the limits you have for yourself. For example: I avoid getting drunk on a first date to ensure I make sound decisions.
- Prioritise what is important for you. For example: I changed jobs to reduce commute time to spend more time with my family.
- Protect your physical and emotional safety. For example: I won't continue to have sex with you if you don't use a condom.
- Define who you are and what algins with your identity/ values. For example: I am available to help you five days a week, but I need some privacy and alone time to take care of my own needs.

Table 8.1 shows some forms healthy and unhealthy boundaries can take. Do you recognise any of them in your interaction with others? (Ray, 2021)

HOW TO IDENTIFY BOUNDARIES

When children feel protected and secure, they begin to understand that certain actions are not acceptable, such as violating someone's physical or emotional well-being, taking something without consent or refusing to engage in activities that make them feel unsafe. However, if we experienced situations where our safety was threatened during our early years, particularly by those who were supposed to protect us, it can be challenging for us to identify and assert our own personal boundaries and rights (Ray, 2021).

Table 8.1 Recognizing healthy and unhealthy boundaries

Healthy boundaries	Unhealthy boundaries
Based on trust and progressive intimacy as trust grows (emotionally and physically)	Trusting everyone or trusting no one
Advocating for personal values and needs	Not expressing and advocating personal values and needs
Identifying and defending your boundaries when someone attempts to cross them	Not knowing your boundaries or not acting to reinforce them when they are crossed
Trusting your decisions	Not trusting your decisions or letting others make decisions for you
Trusting your intuition	Not connecting with or trusting your intuition
Knowing your own identity and what's important to you	Prioritising your life based on what someone else wants from you instead of your values
Maintaining realistic expectations of others	Expecting others to fulfil your every need and know what you want (even when you don't know them yourself)
Communicating your boundaries assertively	Communicating your boundaries passively, passive-aggressively or aggressively
Saying no when required	Not being able to say no when required
Adjusting your boundaries as required when having a negative experience	Closing yourself completely off to all connections and relationships because your boundaries have been crossed in the past

Worksheet 8.1 Where do your boundaries come from?

Spend some time reflecting on the following questions to identify where and what you learnt about boundaries.

- How have you learnt what your boundaries are? Think about the messages you received from the significant adults in your childhood.

- As a child what were you rewarded for? What were you disciplined for?

- How were these patterns helpful or unhelpful?

- How has your participation in formal settings (school, university, work, church, etc.) shaped your boundaries?

HOW DO I KNOW IF MY BOUNDARIES ARE WORKING?

Identifying whether your boundaries are working is important in understanding whether you need to make any adjustments in your relationship with others. You know your boundaries are working if (Ray, 2021):

- Others respect your time, energy, money, assistance and love.
- You know you what your needs and values are, and you feel confident in making decisions about how to prioritise your personal resources.
- You can communicate your boundaries effectively, even if it may be uncomfortable, and reinforce them when they are violated.
- You can recognise when your boundaries are aligned and when they are crossed.
- You understand which boundaries are flexible and contextual and which are deliberately fixed, and you reinforce them accordingly.
- You know when to adjust your boundaries.
- You are willing to adjust your boundaries, but not so rigidly that it prevents others from connecting with you.

IMPACT OF CHILDHOOD EXPERIENCES ON ADULTHOOD BOUNDARIES

Our capacity to set boundaries is built on internal models or blueprints we have for how to relate to others. These mental models reflect our sense of self-worth and expectations for how others will treat us. When a child's needs are overlooked by the trusted adults in their life, they may develop a sense of insecurity in close relationships and may avoid them as a form of protection. These narratives shape our mental models and unconscious behaviours in adulthood (Ray, 2021).

Because our childhood experiences deeply influence our perceptions of self-worth and boundaries, any negative messages we internalise can have a significant impact on how we interact with others as adults (Kerns et al., 2001). Reflect on what was expected of you as a child even when it made you feel unsafe (for example, to face the bullies at school alone 'to learn to stand up on your own feet' or kiss and hug people when you didn't want to 'out of respect for adults'). Did your parents and caregivers parent from a place of 'do as I say not as I do?' or did they role model what was expected of you?

As we discussed in the Emotional Intelligence section, we learn how to respond to our own and other people's emotional needs based on how our parents or caregivers responded to our emotions. If we weren't encouraged to express, process and regulate our emotions and instead were reinforced for people-pleasing, feeling guilty for having emotions or told we were too much or shamed for boundaries we tried to assert, then we may not know how to do that for ourselves. The result is deeply rooted beliefs about our self-worth and sense of boundaries which we don't think about or question and keep repeating as long as we don't review or adjust them.

Worksheet 8.2   Identifying your boundaries (Ray, 2021)

The following questions can help you identify where your boundaries are and what feels authentic for you. There are no right or wrong answers.

- Do you feel energised by spending time with others or alone? (You can assign a percentage to each.)

- What brings you joy?

- What makes you sad?

- What are your strengths?

- What are your weaknesses?

- What are you proud of? What do these things tell you about yourself?

- When faced with a problem, how do you go about solving them?

- When you are frustrated how do you generally respond?

- How do you recover from making a mistake?

- How do you respond when your boundaries are crossed?

- How would someone know that you care about them?

- How would someone else know that you were unhappy with them?

- If you were being your authentic (or ideal) self, what would you be doing (or not doing)?

- Do you believe you are in control of your destiny or that fate is in control of the outcome of your life?

- When going through a tough time, do you prefer to talk about things with another person or process things alone?

- Do you prefer to plan or be spontaneous?

- Are you comfortable with commitments or do you prefer to be uncommitted?

- What are your dealbreakers in relationships (romantic or otherwise)?

- How do you like to be shown love and care?

Worksheet 8.3 Healthy messages for boundary building (Ray, 2021)

Here is a list of some helpful messages you can convey to your child about self-worth and boundaries. Remember, we communicate more effectively via actions than just verbal communication. Think about how you can convey these messages in your daily interactions.

It was great that you tried _____ today.

I've got your back.

Mistakes don't define you.

You are loved.

Your contribution to the family by doing _____ is valuable.

You make a difference by _____.

It's time to let go of _____. It is no longer serving me/us.

I forgive you.

I believe in you.

Comparing yourself with _____ is not helpful.

_____'s reactions to your boundaries is not your responsibility.

I respect your boundaries.

I acknowledge you for doing hard things like _____ and _____.

I admire you for recognising and respecting other people's boundaries.

How to set healthy boundaries
In her book *Setting Boundaries*, Dr Rebecca Ray introduces the model LIMITS as a tool to go about setting healthy boundaries and reinforcing them.

> L—Leader
>
> I—Identify the boundary
>
> M—Make the boundaries known
>
> I—Introduce consequences
>
> T—Take a stand
>
> S—Status check

LEADER

The concept of the Inner Leader as defined by Dr Ray is our authentic self. Before setting a boundary make sure you are connected with the Inner Leader (authentic self) and operating from a place of values and authenticity rather than a place of fear. Refer to the Identifying Values section to connect with what is important for you deep down.

IDENTIFY THE BOUNDARY

- Is the boundary internal or external? Is it an internal boundary you are setting for yourself or is it a boundary you are setting for others?
- What is the function of the boundary? Is it to protect your time, energy, love or other resources? Is it to keep you safe? Is it to maintain your dignity and rights? Is it to ensure you are living based on your values?

Being clear about what the boundary is and what you want it to do can help you communicate it more effectively with others.

MAKE THE BOUNDARY KNOWN

If the boundary is internal, it may be the case of thinking about it with yourself. You could also write them down in a journal or tell a trusted person about them so that you have accountability. If the boundary is between you and another person, communicate it clearly.

INTRODUCE CONSEQUENCES

Think about the consequences if the boundary is being crossed. You may choose to communicate this with the other person at this stage or not. If there are no clear consequences for the boundary being violated they can get confused and blurred.

STATUS CHECK

Check the status of your boundaries. Are they working the way you want them to?

COMMUNICATING YOUR BOUNDARIES

Communicating assertively means advocating for your own rights and needs without violating the rights of others. Using active listening skills as well as clear and firm communication helps you advocate for yourself in a way that is assertive but compassionate, without giving up your own power (passive communication) or blaming and threatening the other person (aggressive communication) or underhandedly expressing anger (passive-aggressive communication).

You can use the following scripts to communicate about your needs and rights. These statements allow you to take responsibility for your feelings and communicate the impact the other person's behaviour has on you and what you need to restore the situation to one of mutual respect.

When _____, I feel _____ (because _____). What I need is _____.

Or

I think your intention was _____.

The impact on me was _____.

What I need is _____.

Here are a couple of examples:

"I don't enjoy this sexual position because it reminds me of a difficult experience I had in the past. In order for me to enjoy sex, I need to avoid that position."

"When you grope me to initiate sex without asking if I am in the mood, I feel disrespected. I need you to verbally check-in with me when you are interested in sex. I find it much more arousing and respectful."

"When I ask you for help around the house and you say you don't have time, I feel frustrated because house chores are mutual responsibilities. What I need is a plan to divide the house chores equally."

Role-modelling
Children learn more from what parents do and less from what they say. Children observe and copy our behaviours. By our own behaviour, by the way in which we express our emotions or solve our conflicts or relate to our partner, we have a great influence on children's behaviour. Our actions guide the social, emotional and relational development of the children and ensure the framework for building healthy sexuality. We teach our children to cooperate and to solve a conflict with another child or to express their anger in a healthy manner by constantly practising the behaviours we want them to learn, during real-life situations and not by explaining things or giving 'advice'.

The most significant relationship education that children receive from their environment about relationships is from their primary caregivers. The way you talk with your partner and about them when they are not present has an enormous impact on the way your child will relate to their future partner/s. As we discussed the things we talk about or not talk about shape the way children view and feel about sexuality and intimacy. So, by modelling the kindness we want to see from our children we give them a template to follow. I think it is also very powerful to tell our children stories of our own experiences. When did we get heartbroken? When did we make a mistake and learn from it (Kogan, 2012)?

Vulnerability

Vulnerability is an essential component of any healthy and fulfilling sexual or romantic relationship. When we allow ourselves to be vulnerable with our partners, we open ourselves up to deeper emotional connections, greater intimacy and a more profound sense of trust. Vulnerability requires us to let go of our emotional defences, allowing ourselves to be seen and understood by our partners in a way that can be both empowering and frightening.

In a sexual context, vulnerability means being able to communicate our desires, boundaries and needs with our partners openly. This can include sharing our sexual fantasies, expressing our insecurities or concerns about our bodies, and being honest about our feelings before, during and after sex. By doing so, we create a space for mutual understanding and respect, allowing our partners to better meet our needs and desires.

In a romantic context, vulnerability means being able to share our fears, hopes and dreams with our partners. It means being able to talk about our past experiences, our struggles and our vulnerabilities without fear of judgement or rejection. Vulnerability also involves being able to listen to our partners, to acknowledge their emotions and to be there for them when they need us.

Without vulnerability, our relationships can become stagnant, distant and unfulfilling. It is only through taking the risk to be vulnerable that we can experience the full depth and richness of our emotional and physical connections with our partners. So if you want to build a healthy and happy sexual or romantic relationship, be willing to be vulnerable and allow your partner to do the same.

One of the common reasons people come to seek therapy is when they do not know how to communicate with their partners about what they want or do not want. It is difficult for them to be vulnerable.

Vulnerability can even play a role in the way we experience sexual pleasure. A study in the UK showed that 80% of sexually active heterosexual women reported that they had faked orgasm in half of their sexual encounters! Although the reason for this is multifaceted (for example, the narrow understanding of sex and orgasm and that generally a sexual encounter is considered over when the man has an orgasm), but for some people (especially women) receiving sexual pleasure makes them feel vulnerable. Being able to be in the moment and willing to surrender to the sensations to enjoy sexual pleasure and potential orgasm can make them feel very raw or self-conscious about how they look when they experience pleasure (Gunsaullus, 2019).

Sometimes people 'perform' sex rather than experience it. This is when they think it is expected of them to perform in a certain way. So, people who sexually perform are likely limiting themselves in their sexual experience to what they think is appropriate and expected. Secondly, they prioritise performing for a partner over feeling their own embodied sensations and pleasure.

So, the bottom line is no one is perfect, and it is okay to show our imperfections, to acknowledge when we make mistakes or do not know the answer to questions or look awkward, silly or vulnerable. The way we handle our lack of knowledge, ambiguity and discomfort can be the difference between living a life based on the expectations of others or leading a rewarding and genuine life based on our principles.

PARENTS' Q&A

Table 8.2 Parents' Q&A

Parent's question	My response
How can I respect my child's sense of agency when I have to do necessary things which they don't like or even hate, such as changing nappies or putting warm clothes on?	The aim in our interaction with children is to minimise the sense of helplessness and maximise respect and agency. Here are some strategies you can use: Connect & slow down—If you treat nappy change or getting dressed as a chance to connect and enjoy your child, they are more likely to enjoy the connection and therefore cooperate with the activity. If you rush through it like it's something unpleasant, they will react as if they are being held down and subjected to something unpleasant, which, indeed, it can be when you rush a nappy change or pulling down that tight turtleneck.
	Treat your child with respect—Even though babies don't understand our words, they feel the difference when they are treated with respect. So instead of just scooping them up, move slowly and explain what's happening. Even tiny babies understand tone of voice. After a while they have better associations with nappy changes and don't build up as much resistance. Create predictability—The other thing you do is to create a sense of predictability. This is especially important for babies and toddlers who don't understand verbal language yet. Change their nappy and clothes in the same room or spot, tell them before you pick them up what is going to happen. You can also count down three to before you start the process. After a while they can predict what is going to happen, which minimises feelings of helplessness (when combined with other strategies mentioned).
	Help them transition—If they are in the middle of playing with their favourite toy, help them take the object to the changing table: "Let's drive your car to the changing table." Empathise—In a calm voice tell them you understand their point of view: "You don't like nappy change time. You like to run around and play. It is hard for you to stay still."

Healthy boundaries

Parent's question	My response
	Make it something to look it forward to—make a collection of their favourite toys/objects and make them available only during nappy change time. Change the environment—get curious about what about changing nappies or wearing warm clothes that your child doesn't like. Is it the cold wipes? Get a wet wipe warmer. Is it the tight neck of the sweater? Buy some button-up jumpers. Sometimes it is easier than it seems. Most important of all, don't make nappy changing into a battle. No child should regularly be held down while their clothing is pulled off or being changed. That's not a good foundation for learning consent. No one approach will always work, so you'll have to mix and match and be willing to get creative.
How do I respond when I see my three-year-old touch her genitals in public?	Young children naturally explore their body parts, including their genitals, and it is a developmentally typical behaviour. It is your job to help them understand when it is socially acceptable to touch their genitals. If your child starts to play with their genitals in a public place, gently tell them: "Honey, I know if feels good to touch your penis/vulva. But we only touch our genitals in a private place like in the bedroom or bathroom." If the child is too young to understand verbal communication, find something else that feels soothing or pleasurable for them to do. Hand them their comforter or favourite toy or pick them up and give them a hug. Treating body parts as 'rude' or shameful has very negative effects on children's sense of self and sexuality.
How can I support my teenager when he is going through a breakup?	A breakup is a good opportunity to teach children about emotions, loss and grief, love and relationships. Acknowledge that it can be difficult to experience a heartbreak (if that is what your child is experiencing) and that grief is a process that most people go through when a relationship ends (you can refer to the following 'Stages of grief' for more details). Give your child permission to feel their feelings (sadness, anger, disappointment, despair, etc.). Remind them that things will get better and they will experience love and joy again, that a breakup is part of our experience of being a human. If you did have a similar experience when you were their age, share your story with them. Encourage them to process their feelings by taking actions: talking to you or a trusted person, journaling, running, swimming,

(Continued)

Table 8.2 Continued

Parent's question	My response
	playing music. If your child shows signs of depression over time (lack of appetite, isolation, aggression, self-harm, suicidal thoughts, insomnia, etc.) do seek support from a mental health professional.
	Stages of grief after a breakup (Kubler-Ross, 1969): It is important to know that grief is a very personal experience. It's not very neat or linear, and it doesn't follow any time lines or schedules. Everyone grieves differently, but there are some commonalities in the stages of grief experienced by many people. The stages of grief after a breakup can occur all at once, or at varying times during the process of letting go.
	1. Denial
	Denial is our brain's automatic response to unwanted news. Denial gives our mind and heart time to adjust to the new situation. In the denial phase we may think that our significant other is coming back. Everybody spends different amounts of time in the denial phase.
	2. Anger and confusion
	The person who is on the receiving end of a breakup may feel genuinely confused as why their partner ended the relationship. When a breakup happens, the partner on the receiving end of it can react in angry outbursts: "You can't do this to me!" or "I won't let you leave me."
	3. Bargaining
	The person is willing to do anything to avoid accepting it's over. They would be a better, more attentive partner. Everything that's been wrong, they will make right. The thought of being without the significant other is so intolerable that they are willing to do anything by winning their partner back, at any cost.
	4. Acknowledgement and grieving
	This stage begins when the person finally admits that the relationship is over. It is in this stage that grief is felt deeply and sometimes intensely. While both/all parties experience a level of grief, the person who was at the receiving end of the breakup may experience it more deeply in the form of rejection or abandonment.
	5. Acceptance and hope
	As acceptance deepens, hope for a better future grows—from the belief that you can save a failing relationship to the possibility that you just might be okay without your ex.

Healthy boundaries

Parent's question	My response
What do I do if my child says they are not the gender we thought they were?	Parental support plays a significant role in trans and gender-diverse children and young people. A study in 2016 showed that trans children who were supported by their parents had similar mental health outcomes as a cisgender control group (Olson et al., 2016). Research shows that transgender youth experience higher rates of depression and suicidal thoughts compared to cisgender peers. Some people interpret this as being transgender inherently increases the likelihood of experiencing mental health issues. However, the reality is that the level of support a young person receives is a more significant factor in determining their mental health outcomes, rather than their gender identity. So, how can you support your child? During the process of a child coming out as transgender, parents and family members may experience a wide range of emotions, including confusion, fear, love and protectiveness. Seeking support from a qualified professional, such as a sexologist or psychologist with experience in gender identity, can help navigate these uncertainties. Trust your child's intuitions. Being transgender or any other gender identity is an internal experience. Only the person can say what gender they identify with and therefore what their gender identity is. Your child might be able to explain to you what's going on with them, but they might also not have the words. Tell your child that you love them and you accept them, even if you don't understand. Thank them for telling you, because it can be a huge deal that they've told you about this, especially if they're not sure if you're going to be accepting or not. Trust their intuition and the needs they express. For instance, they may have specific language that they would like you to use. If your child was assigned male by the doctor when they were born but they say they identify as a girl, they may ask you to use she, her and hers as their pronouns and treat them just as you would any other girl. Do your best to respect their wishes. Creating a safe space in your home where your child can freely explore their gender identity without judgement is crucial. They may not always be safe to do so in the world, so it's crucial that they know there is a safe space. Carve out a little safe haven where they can play and explore and be free without the judgement they might experience in the world outside.

(Continued)

Table 8.2 Continued

Parent's question	My response
	Stay flexible. Childhood is a time when all of us explore our gender identities, regardless of whether we're transgender or not. So staying flexible and allowing them the space to express themselves is important. Know that you're probably going to make mistakes, and that is okay. Approach it with curiosity and the intention of supporting your child. Focus on your connection with them and their sense of safety. If you use the wrong language for them or say something that doesn't feel right to them, just apologise and work on correcting yourself in the future. Get curious about your child's inner world and experiences. It can be a difficult time for you and your family, so do connect with your support network and self-care strategies and do seek support for your own mental well-being.

REFERENCE LIST

Gunsaullus, J. (2019). *From madness to mindfulness: Reinventing sex for women* (1st ed., p. 28). Cleis Press.

Kerns, K. A., Aspelmeier, J. E., Gentzler, A. L., & Grabill, C. M. (2001). Parent-child attachment and monitoring in middle childhood. *Journal of Family Psychology, 15*(1), 69–81. https://doi.org/10.1037/0893-3200.15.1.69

Kogan, J. (2012). Brené Brown: Be the adult you want your children to be. *The Washington Post*. Retrieved May 28, 2021, from https://www.washingtonpost.com/blogs/on-parenting/post/brene-brown-be-the-adult-you-want-your-children-to-be/2012/10/04/b5bdbd9c-0ca6-11e2-a310-2363842b7057_blog.html

Kubler-Ross, E. (1969). *On death and dying*. Routledge.

Olson, K. R., Durwood, L., DeMeules, M., & McLaughlin, K. A. (2016). Mental health of transgender children who are supported in their identities. *Pediatrics, 137*(3), e20153223. https://doi.org/10.1542/peds.2015-3223

Ray, R. (2021). *Setting boundaries*. Pan Macmillan Australia.

Part 3
Topics to talk about with children

CHAPTER 9

What topics to talk about?

So far, we have discussed the skills necessary for young people to make sound decisions about their sexual lives, manage uncomfortable feelings and situations, and develop fundamental skills for fulfilling relationships. Hopefully, by now you are feeling more prepared and confident to provide sexuality education to your children. But what topics should you cover? What language is appropriate to use? How can you increase the chance of your message being received by your young one? In this chapter I have included some topics and suggestions for language which are the foundations of current comprehensive sexuality education.

However, I would like to acknowledge that we live in a world where information and our understanding of the world is constantly updated and expanded. So, it would be impractical if I told you about the latest research about sexually transmitted infections, contraception or even gender and sexual orientation. However, I can share with you some broad areas that have maintained importance and relevance in the field of sexuality over the years, which I believe can guide your decision-making on the topic.

A NOTE ON LANGUAGE

The attitude we have to our bodies and sex are closely tied up in language. Sadly, a lot of shame is embodied within many languages about sex and even body parts. Some examples are:

- English: 'rude' parts, 'dirty talk', 'walk of shame'
- Persian: 'sharmgah' (place of shame) refence to the pelvis

- German: 'schamhaar' (shame-hair) reference to pubic hair
- Spanish: 'partes pudendas' (shameful parts) reference to genitals

The less confidently we discuss our bodies, the more difficult it will be to embrace our sexuality and pleasure and to ensure we have safe and enjoyable sexual experiences. Being able to accurately identify body parts opens up the ability to communicate our needs and desires and describe things accurately if we are seeking help or communicating with our partner/s.

Sometimes we use 'secret language' to communicate about sex and sexuality. This is usually to cover up for our own discomfort. When we talk to children about their 'rude parts', 'private parts' or 'down there' we are using indirect or 'secret' language. When we refer to periods as TOM (time of the month), 'the curse' or 'a visit from the aunty' we are using secret language and are very likely to miss out on great opportunities to have important conversations about puberty, bodies, gender and sexuality. Using secret language can add to the stigma of talking about sexuality and can make it difficult for our children to reach out to us when they need to (Vernacchio, 2014).

Even small children pick up that there are certain body parts that we use a 'special language' for or don't talk about at all. Since young children don't understand why, they can develop feelings of shame, confusion or fear about their genitals or about sexuality in general (Vernacchio, 2014). "But what if they say the words out loud in front of others?" is what many people who use indirect language ask. But what is the worst case that can happen? The adults in the room will feel embarrassed. Is this worth damaging our children's healthy relationship with their body and sexuality? Also, when children learn certain language to refer to their body parts it can be an additional barrier to talk with their parents about sexuality. Many children don't find a way to replace that language with something more suitable when they are older and believe me, I have had clients who didn't let their parents know they were suffering from an infection because they didn't know what language to use. It was too awkward and shameful for them.

THE PLACE

Sometimes the place we choose to have conversations about sexuality can have a lasting impact on our kids. One of my clients, Laura, who was experiencing pain with intercourse told me about her first exposure to sexuality education, which she recalled as "an extremely painful emotional experience". Her mother had told her to go to her parents' bedroom, which was a place she would usually be sent when she was in trouble or if there was news about someone's death. Laura remembers sitting there in cold sweat waiting for the bad news to come. And to her surprise her mother told her: "You are now a big girl and should know about women's business." Although there was no punishment or news about death, the feelings associated with that conversation remained with Laura for years and was one of the contributing factors to her sexual pain.

As I mentioned before sexuality education is not one 'big talk' but lots of small conversations throughout years. Conversations about sexuality are best received and reciprocated when they happen organically. A song on the radio, a social media post, a scene in a movie can all be used as opportunities to have these conversations and educate your kids about healthy sexuality. We already do this, but this is a reminder to use these opportunities mindfully and intentionally. Conversations about sexuality are more successful when it flows naturally rather than creating a special place for a serious talk.

When your toddler plays with their genitals is a good time to start talking about sexuality (naming body parts, for example), or when your tween daughter talks about being too thin or too fat what you say can influence the way she thinks and feels about her body and her sexuality. When your teenage son is reading magazines with content that divides the world into stereotypical categories of men and women, you can affirm or challenge the notion. These are all conversations about sexuality, and you can take advantage of these moments.

Here are some conversation starters if you are wondering how it could look in practice:

> "What did you think about the way Rose responded to Jackson's proposal? Most often men propose to women in movies, what do you think about women proposing to men?"
>
> "I was thinking about what Aunt Layla said yesterday about boys being boys. What do you think she meant by that?"
>
> "What kind of relationship would you like to have in the future? Have you ever thought about it?"
>
> "Can I tell you about the time Grandma and Grandpa met? It is a funny and lovely story!"
>
> "Do you know when your mum and I were dating I felt so anxious I couldn't sleep much?"
>
> "What is your biggest worry when it comes to dating?"
>
> "Some people think everyone *needs* a partner to be happy. What do you think?"
>
> "What do you think this song is referring to?"
>
> "I wonder what this ad says about how young men should behave."
>
> "Have you noticed there is little about other genders in the movies we watch? Where do you think we can find more diverse movies?"

Most often these conversations help kids have a better understanding of their parent's world view and values without feeling they are being lectured. Asking kids about their opinion and involving them in a conversation also promotes autonomy and respect. Most teens feel more connected to their parents when they know the parents are interested in the same topics they are interested in. When you incorporate sexuality in everyday conversation you are sending an important message to your kids, that sexuality is a normal part of life (Vernacchio, 2014).

IT'S NOT ABOUT SEX

Remember, a lot of sexuality education is not about the act of sex. There are many conversations you can have about sex and sexuality without talking about naked bodies and intercourse. This is particularly important when you have young children. Remember, you are building a healthy frame of reference for their sexuality. Just as I mentioned before any conversation you have about bodies, love, relationships, gender roles, gender expression (including clothing), what it means to be a man, woman, other genders, puberty, communication, empathy are all aspects of sexuality education. Story telling is a wonderful and powerful way of teaching children about the world and themselves. All cultures have the element of storytelling to pass on familial knowledge and values to the next generation (Doucleff, 2021). You can buy books, but you can use your imagination and tell them a simple story about one of the topics previously mentioned. You can even engage your young one to create a story together and along the way you can teach important lessons about values and world views related to sexuality and relationships.

TALK WITH TEACHERS AND YOUR CHILD ABOUT THE CURRENT SEXUAL/RELATIONAL ISSUES AT SCHOOL

Keeping in close contact with young people's experiences is critical in presenting them with information which is of interest and relevance to their life. You can ask your young person or their teacher about relational/sexual issues they encounter in their physical and cyber world and what they think about them. Never underestimate a young person's inner wisdom. Time and time again I have been surprised by the insight young people have and the solutions they come up with when met with validation and curiosity.

ASK QUESTIONS RATHER THAN JUST PRESENTING INFORMATION

For example, instead of saying something like, "there are a few different ways to prevent unintended pregnancy, condoms, pills, IUD, etc.," you could ask "tell me what you have heard about the different types of contraception." This facilitates a conversation rather than a monologue of you presenting information to your child which they may already have.

Consent

The term 'consent' is often associated with sex, but it's much broader than that. It relates to permission and how to show respect for ourselves and for other people. It also includes how to set boundaries, communicate effectively and display empathy.

It is crucial to consider what consent means before looking at when and how we teach our children about it (Rare, 2020):

- Consent is about communication, agency and respect. It is an essential part of relationships.
- Consent in a sexual context is pleasure-focused and should be given enthusiastically.
- Consent can be withdrawn or altered at any time.
- Consent is about specific activities and is not a blanket rule.
- Most often the teaching we/our children receive about consent is how to protect ourselves from danger, and therefore there is a lot of emphasis on communicating what we don't want. But in most relationships consent is about increasing pleasure and having a good time, so

knowing what we want and communicating that with our partner is an important part of navigating consent.

Teaching consent starts from a very young age. We can normalise asking our children for consent when we want to touch them. Imagine you lived in a world where most people were larger in size than you and they told you what you could eat, what clothes you could wear and when you had to sleep, and these large people touched you (in a loving way) as they pleased even when you didn't like it or when you protested by screaming. This is what the world feels like for our children. Children communicate with us about what they like and don't like all the time, even babies do. By respecting our children's needs and desire for touch we are teaching them they have autonomy over their body and they have the right to get upset when it is violated.

What does this look like in practice? If your child is an infant or a toddler, pay attention to their body language. Do they relax in your arms, when you kiss them and touch them or do they tense up and look uncomfortable? If they don't seem to enjoy it, put them back down and verbalise that realisation: "you don't like me to pick you up right now, so I am putting you back down here." Babies may not have the cognitive capacity to understand verbal communication, but they do understand tone of voice, emotions and our actions. This verbal communication also teaches them an important regulation skill which becomes very important to deal with stress later in life. Studies in child emotional development show that parents who get curious about the child's needs and internal processes and respond accordingly help the child develop skills for self-awareness and self-regulation (Kerns et al., 2001). When a baby cries, most parents intuitively say something like: "What is going on, Sweetie? Does your tummy hurt? Let me give it a rub. Let's try this position." Or when the baby is smiling you may say something like: "That big poop made you really happy, didn't it?" Throughout time children learn to get curious about their own emotional state and the cause for it. For example, when they feel sad, they can identify it and get curious about the reason they feel that way. People who have had experiences of neglect or abuse in childhood lack this fundamental skill for self-regulation. They cannot identify what they are feeling and therefore feel helpless and desperate because they cannot influence or regulate their emotional state.

If you have older children, you can teach consent by letting them know when you want to touch them and respect their wish if they refuse. Instead of pulling them in your arms and squeezing them with affection when they obviously don't like it, you can let them know what you wish for and wait for them to initiate the touch or stop as soon as you see signs of discomfort. Our intention as parents, grandparents, aunties and uncles is to express love and affection, but when it is done in a way that doesn't consider the needs and the pleasure of the child, the impact is internalisation of this implicit message: "Adults have authority over my body. My body is for their enjoyment and I can't do anything to stop it." I think it is clear how this schema or thought pattern can lead to feelings of helplessness, hopelessness and despair when it comes to abuse. You can also give children agency over what is age-appropriate, like what snack to have, or what to read at story time.

During Christmas time if you walk past any Santa stand you will most likely hear at least one child crying in fear of Santa and a parent asking their kid to just sit on Santa's knee for a photo. What most parents don't realise is that unknowingly they are asking their child to override their feelings and their gut intuition about safety. It's overriding their ability to express consent and to trust their instincts from a very young age.

Other ways of teaching young children about consent are teaching them how to ask others for permission and how to give permission and voice their emotions. Violet, a four-year-old girl, loves hugging other kids. But not all children enjoy being interrupted in the middle of a game to be hugged. Luke, Violet's teacher, teaches her how to ask for permission. "You can ask Sam if she would like a hug now or later. You can save the hug for her for when you and her both want it." Violet now has a bank full of deposited hugs and happily hugs other kids when they are interested.

You can even teach children about empathy and consent through their interactions with other kids or even animals. When Janice bought Jackson her six-year-old a puppy for Christmas, she taught Jackson how to pay attention to the animal's body language to understand when it wants to be held, touched or left alone. "When Salty make this noise, it means she doesn't want to be touched anymore." Another example of teaching young children about consent through play is teaching your child to play games that are enjoyable for everyone. If you hear one of them say "If you don't play with me, I won't be your friend anymore," you can intervene and model: "It looks like Jessy doesn't want to play this game right now. You can choose something you both like or you can do two different things separately. Jessy, it's okay that you don't want to play. Let Samira know if you change your mind."

These early interactions with parents, other adults and peers also teach children important lessons about consensual touch, pleasure and respect. If you are a 17-year-old who has been treated all your childhood and teenage years as if your voice and your autonomy didn't matter, how likely is that you would understand real-life applications of consent in sexual and romantic relationships when you learn about it at school (if you learn about it at all).

Children need to learn they have a choice in how they react, so when they're older they don't resort to blaming someone else's behaviour for their actions. In various situations take the opportunity to teach your child "You may not be happy about it, but you have a choice about that. How you respond to that is your choice." By acknowledging children's agency from an early age and supporting it throughout their childhood, messages about sexual consent can be more effectively reinforced and ingrained as they grow older.

If you have teens and have not done the aforementioned things when they were young, don't panic. You are not a bad parent, and your child is not broken. We all bring up our children with best intentions and the information we have available to us in that point in time. You can still do a lot and teach a lot about consent. It is never too late.

It is important to understand that during puberty and the transition to adulthood, teenagers tend to establish a distinct identity from their parents, which is a natural and healthy part of growing up. As a result, teenagers typically seek autonomy and independence more than children of other ages. By respecting their sense of autonomy and independence and providing a safe space for them for self-exploration, you teach them you respect their need for autonomy and a sense of individuality. Although teenagers look a lot more like adults than pre-teens and young children, their brains have not fully developed and their needs for physical touch by parents is as important as other children. Make sure you don't discontinue hugging them and expressing physical affection just because they have reached a certain age. Let them know you enjoy the touch, but don't initiate or continue when they say no.

One of the gaps in the current education about consent is the tendency to oversimplify asking and giving consent. 'No means no' is at the core of most education about consent. That is not incorrect. No does mean no. However, this oversimplification fails to recognise the nuance of how we tend to say no to things. Very rarely in life do we say 'no' to things we don't like to do. We usually use other ways of communicating the fact that we don't want to (Rare, 2021):

- Deflection: "I don't really feel like it right now." Or "I've got a different suggestion."
- Excuses: "I've got a headache." Or "I can't. I am too busy right now."
- Postponing: "I'll do it tomorrow." Or "Ask me another time."
- Using polite language: "I prefer not to, if you don't mind." Or "That's a lovely offer, but I'm happy doing this instead."

We may also use negotiation:

- "I hate vacuuming. Would you do it? I will do the dishes."
- "I can't call him right now, but I will put a reminder in my calendar to call him tomorrow."
- "I don't feel very sexy right now. Can I hold you while you touch yourself?"

Negotiation and compromise are important parts of consent and relationships, but you should always be okay with the outcome of the negotiation. Negotiation when used with empathy, compassion and active listening skills is one of the most effective tools in healthy relationships.

Another point about consent is that it is not one definitive conversation, a yes or no conclusion. There should be an initial conversation ("I really feel like giving you a big hug right now. Is that okay?") followed by paying attention to the other's body language and non-verbal communication as well verbal check-ins ("how does this feel for you?") with opportunities to continue enthusiastically consenting or changing/adjusting/negotiating or withdrawing some or all of consent. Communicating consent is something that happens throughout a (sexual) interaction, not just before it.

Talk to your teen about what consent is and what it means to them. Teenagers are old enough to understand some nuances of relationships. You can discuss how adding alcohol and drugs to the picture could cloud consent or when the other person's verbal language doesn't match their body language or tone of voice. You can also talk about power dynamics in relationships and how that can affect meaningful consent (for example, age difference, a person in a supervisory role, having a disability, etc.) Books and television shows can provide great learning opportunities, where you can ask your child what they think about what's happening or what the characters are feeling.

Keep in mind that no message is stronger than actions. If you have a partner, how do you communicate with them? Do you role model asking for consent in front of your children? It doesn't have to be about sexual topics. It could be as simple as asking for their permission to share a photo of them on social media.

CONSENT AT EVERY AGE (GILLIS ET AL., 2021)

Age 0–5 years:

1. Teach your child to ask permission before touching or embracing a playmate. Use language such as "Darling, let's ask Sarah if she would like to hug bye-bye." If Sarah says no to this request, cheerfully tell your child, "That's okay! Let's wave bye-bye to Sarah and blow her a kiss."
2. Help create empathy within your child by explaining how something they have done may have hurt someone. For example, "I know you wanted that toy, but when you hit Jack, it hurt him and he feels sad." Encourage your child to imagine how they might feel if Jack had hit them instead. This can be done with a loving tone and a big hug so the child doesn't feel ashamed or embarrassed.
3. Teach your kids that "no" and "stop" are important words and should be honoured. One way to explain this may be, "Sarah said 'no', and when we hear 'no' we always stop what we're doing immediately." Also teach your child that their no's are to be honoured. Explain that just like we always stop doing something when someone says no, that our friends need to always stop when we say no, too. If a friend doesn't stop when we say no, then we need to think about whether or not we feel good, and safe, playing with them. If not, it's okay to choose not to play. Role model stopping when you hear your child say no to touch.
4. Encourage your child to read facial expressions and body language. Charade-style guessing games with expressions are a great way to teach children how to read body language.
5. Never force a child to hug, touch or kiss anybody, for any reason. If Grandma is demanding a kiss and your child is resistant, offer alternatives by saying something like, "Would you rather give Grandma a high-five or blow her a kiss, maybe?"

6. Encourage children to wash their own genitals during bath time. Of course parents have to help sometimes, but explaining to your daughter that her vulva is important and that she needs to take care of it is a great way to help encourage body pride and a sense of ownership of their own body.
7. Give them the opportunity to say yes or no in everyday choices, too. Let your child choose clothing and have a say in what they wear, what they play or how they do their hair. Obviously, there are times when you have to step in (a −10 °C winter day when your child wants to wear a summer dress would be one of those times!), but help them understand that you heard their voice and that it mattered to you, but that you want to keep them safe and healthy. "You don't want to wear a jumper. I get that. My job is to keep you safe, and sometimes I have to make decisions for you that are not comfortable. You can choose which jumper to wear today or you can put the jumper in your bag and when you feel cold put it on" (refer to page xx for managing conflicts when it comes to nappy changing or particular clothes).
8. Allow your child to talk about their body in any way they want, without shame. Teach them the correct words for their genitals, and make yourself a safe place for talking about bodies. Say, "I'm so glad you asked me that!" If you don't know the answer to a particular question say, "I'm glad you're asking me about this, but I don't know the answer. I will look it up and we can talk about it later." and make sure you follow up with them when you say you will.
9. Talk about "gut feelings" or instincts. Explain that sometimes things make us feel weird or scared or yucky and we don't know why. Teach them that this "belly voice" is important to pay attention to and that if they ever have a gut feeling that is confusing, they can always come to you for help in sorting through their feelings and making decisions.

Ages 5–12

1. Teach them that the way their body is changing is great but can sometimes be confusing. The way you talk about these changes—whether it's loose teeth or pimples and

pubic hair—will show your willingness to talk about other subjects and normalises changes in their body.
2. Encourage them to talk about what feels good and what doesn't. "Do you like to be tickled? Do you like to be held tight? What else? What doesn't feel good?" Provide the space for your child to talk about anything else that comes to mind.
3. Teach kids how to use safe words during play, and help them negotiate a safe word to use with their friends. This is helpful because many kids like to disappear deep into their pretend worlds and characters, such as playing war games where someone gets captured, or putting on a stage play where characters may be arguing. In cases like this, saying no may be part of the play, so they need to have one word that will stop all activity. Maybe it's a silly one like "peanut butter" or a serious one like "I really mean it!", or even "safe word". Whatever works for all of them. If someone uses the safe word the play needs to stop to understand what is going wrong and if necessary get help for the person. Teach them never to use the safe word as a joke. It is only for when you need others to stop the play.
4. Teach them to stop their play every once in a while to check in with one another. Teach them to take a moment out of their play every so often, to make sure everyone's feeling okay. Role model this in your interactions with other adults and children.
5. Encourage kids to pay attention to each other's facial expressions and body language during play. Most human communication is non-verbal. Other people's tone of voice, body language and facial expression can tell us a lot about their internal state. Helping kids learn these communication skills is fundamental for healthy relationships.
6. Don't tease your child for having crushes or being in love with another child. Whatever they feel is okay. If their friendship with someone else seems like a crush, don't mention it. You can ask them open questions like, "How is your friendship with Hans going?" Give them space to talk about it or choose to keep it private.
7. Teach your child that every person's behaviour can affect others. You can do this in simple ways, anywhere. Teach them to observe how people respond when other people

make noise or litter. Ask them what they think will happen as a result. Will someone else have to clean up the litter? Will someone be scared? Explain to kids how the choices they make affect others and talk about when are good times to be loud and where are good spaces to be messy, etc.

Teenage years

1. Talk about consent. One of the common games that emerges in this age is 'touch games': butt-slapping, boys hitting one another in the genitals and pinching each other's nipples, etc. Having conversations about consent in this context paves the way to teach them about consent in sexual and romantic relationships in the future. Help them understand how they can identify if the other person is enjoying this 'game'. Explain to them that if the other person is not happy or if the touch was uninvited it could be sexual harassment or even assault.
2. Build their self-esteem. In teenage years bullying shifts to specifically target identity, and self-esteem starts to fall around age 13. A survey of mental health and well-being in Australia showed body image as a major concern for more than 30% of teenagers (Mission Australia, 2019). We tend to build up our smaller kids by telling them how great they are. For some reason, sometimes people stop telling their teens all the wonderful aspects of who they are when they reach middle school. But this is actually a very crucial time to be building up our kids' self-esteem, and not just about beauty. Remark to them regularly about their talents, their skills, their kindness, as well as their appearance.
3. Have conversations about relationships Ask questions like, "How do you know whether your partner is ready to kiss you?" or "How do you think you can tell if someone is interested in a relationship with you?"
4. Have open and continuous conversations about healthy sexuality. Teens are thirsty for more information about healthy sexuality. They want to learn, and they will find a way to get information about it. If you are the one providing that information with love, transparency and

consistency they are more likely to come to you than to seek out information from peers and pornography.
5. Convey the following messages about healthy sexuality:
- Consensual sex is a healthy part of life, and I have the right to experience pleasure if and when I choose to.
- Provided they are done consensually, all sexual expressions and practices are valid even if they differ from my own.
- I have the right to take ownership of my body and sexual choices.

REFERENCE LIST

Doucleff, M. (2021). *Hunt, gather, parent: What ancient cultures can Teach us about the lost art of raising happy, helpful little humans.* Simon & Schuster.

Gillis, J., Utt, J., Royse, A., & Schroeder, J. (2021). The healthy sex talk: Teaching kids consent, ages 1–21. Retrieved August 2023, from https://www.talkwithyourkids.org/lets-talk-about/healthy-sex-talk-teaching-kids-consent-ages-1-21.html

Kerns, K. A., Aspelmeier, J. E., Gentzler, A. L., & Grabill, C. M. (2001). Parent-child attachment and monitoring in middle childhood. *Journal of Family Psychology*, 15(1), 69–81. https://doi.org/10.1037/0893-3200.15.1.69

Mission Australia. (2019). *Youth survey report 2019.* https://www.missionaustralia.com.au/publications/youth-survey

Rare, R. (2020). *Sex ed for adults.* Vermilion.

Rare, R. (2021). *Sex ed: A belated guide for adults.* Bloomsbury.

Vernacchio, A. (2014). *For goodness sex: Changing the way we talk to teens about sexuality, values, and health.* HarperCollins.

CHAPTER 10
Provide a balanced and realistic view of sex

Sometimes parents, with good intentions, provide fear-based information to their children, such as "having sex can put you at risk of STIs. Some of them are not treatable and you can even die from them." Or "you don't want to get pregnant at 14, do you? Well, if you have sex there is no guarantee that won't happen. Think about how that can ruin your whole life."

Firstly, information like this can create fear in children about sex. I have seen clients who were unable to engage in sexual activities with their partner due to the messages they continuously received about sex from their environment. These messages often portray sex as dirty and dangerous. If you succeed in making your child scared of having sex, that fear will not magically disappear when they find a loving partner or get married.

Secondly, children are exposed to various sources of information about sex and sexuality, including their peers. Sooner or later, they will receive messages from other sources that sex can be pleasurable and exciting. Coupled with the rise of sexual hormones in their body, they tend to prioritise messages about pleasure and excitement over fear-inducing messages. Additionally, the part of the adolescent brain that assesses risk (the pre-frontal cortex) has yet to develop fully, so they often underestimate the risk even when it is real and probable. Consequently, many adolescents end up having sex to satisfy their curiosity. However, when they need help and guidance, they are unlikely to seek it from their parents because they were initially "warned" by them.

Most forms of sexuality education at their core have some good advice, but by packaging them up with a lot of negative feelings, such as fear, disgust and shame, we often miss those core messages. Even if the content of sex ed is accurate, if it's presented by a teacher who's too embarrassed to talk about it, or if it's loaded with fear-based messages, it can be just as harmful to a young person as the content itself.

Most formal sex education at schools, to date, is still based on heterosexual sex and does not equip young people to navigate consent. It also fails to mention that pleasure is important and valid. Consent is usually presented as a legal requirement to have sex not an important aspect of pleasurable sex.

What we can do as parents is to provide information that is positive, realistic and balanced. Here are some examples of how to reframe fear-based or shaming messages with more positive ones.

Is abstinence-based sexuality education effective? Let's have a look at the research:

> To understand the effectiveness of different approaches to sex ed, a study compared sexual health outcomes for young people in Australia and the Netherlands, where comprehensive sexuality education is taught, and the United States, where abstinence-only education was taught in some states. Researchers tracked rates of HIV and STI transmission, and unintended pregnancies.
>
> The average age of first intercourse was similar in the Netherlands (17.7 years) and Australia (16 years). But sexual health outcomes where abstinence-only programs were taught fell well behind. Teens in the US had an earlier age of first sexual intercourse (15.8), higher rates of pregnancy terminations and higher rates of teen births compared with the other countries in the study. Around 30.4 out of every 1,000 women aged 15 to 17 in the US will give birth.

Provide a balanced and realistic view of sex

Table 10.1 Reframing fear-based and shaming messages with positive alternatives

Common Fear-based/Shaming Messages	Possible Re-frame	Rationale
If you have sex, you'll be labelled as a slut/man-whore.	You have the right to make your own decisions about your body and your relationships. To have an enjoyable experience make sure you feel safe with the person you want to have sex with and remember to communicate with each other about your wants and needs.	Helps young people feel more empowered and confident in their decisions, while also promoting a more inclusive and accepting culture around sexuality.
Don't be embarrassed to buy condoms; pregnancy or an STI are even more embarrassing!	Protecting yourself and your partner is important, and buying condoms is a responsible and mature thing to do. It's important to work through any feelings of embarrassment about buying condoms.	Removes feeling of shame from unintended pregnancy and STIs.
Your first time should be with someone special, or you'll regret it.	Your first time is a personal and individual experience, and it's important to make sure you feel comfortable and ready before engaging in sexual activity. What matters most is that you are making a choice that feels right for you and that you are with a partner you feel safe with.	Removes judgement/shame and emphasises communication.

The Netherlands stands out as having one of the lowest rates of teen pregnancy in the world (2.2 births per 1,000 women aged 15 to 17).

CHAPTER 11
Include pleasure in your conversation about sexuality

Most people grow up with the message that reproduction or procreation is the reason people have sex. Sex is about making babies. Almost all the sexuality education available until now are focused on the biological aspects of sex and risk minimisation. The concept of pleasure, which is a fundamental part of the human experience with links to positive health and well-being outcomes, is largely absent from sex education in most countries around the world (Urban, 2018).

It is important to talk about the pleasure of intimacy and why that is important, and how you develop and maintain intimate relationships. Pleasurable sexual experiences are strongly correlated to overall physical and mental wellbeing, protect against sexual (re)traumatisation and, for most people, have a major impact on their quality of life (University of Amsterdam, 2017).

Pleasure-absent sexuality education reinforces sexual pleasure inequalities in two ways. Firstly, by solely focusing on preventing STIs and pregnancy without mentioning pleasure, there's an implicit message that sex only involves vaginal intercourse and male ejaculation is the central aspect. Secondly, pleasureless sex education neglects to teach individuals how to communicate their desires, which is crucial in preventing sexual violence. It's difficult to consent to something when you don't know what you find pleasurable. Furthermore, it's easier to refuse unwanted behaviour when you feel empowered to say yes to what you do want (Barrett, 2019).

PLEASURE-BASED VERSUS RISK-BASED APPROACH TO SEXUALITY EDUCATION

The current mainstream approach to sexuality education is a risk-based approach. A risk-based approach to sex reinforces fear or shame as the main motivator for people to use sexual protection. For example, when we want to teach about safer sex methods we usually say something like: "if you have sex without a condom, you will get HIV so you'd better use a condom." A pleasure approach focuses on pleasure as a valid and legitimate reason to have sex and that sexuality should not be about fear, shame or stigma, but about happiness, satisfaction and fulfilment. So, a pleasure-based approach to condom use could look like this: "Did you know that if you use a condom plus contraceptive pills you can enjoy sex without having to worry about unintended pregnancies and STIs?"

Table 11.1 Risk-based versus pleasure-based approach to sexuality education

Risk-based approach	Pleasure-based approach	Rationale
	A female condom can help stimulate the clitoris and just like a male condom reduce the risk of STIs. It is important to see which option feels more pleasurable and practical for you and your partner.	Promotes pleasure as a key ingredient for people to practise safer sax and be protected.
If you have sex without a condom you will get HIV.		This reinforces fear or shame as the main motivators for people to use protection and focuses messages solely on HIV as an unintended consequence of sexual activity.
	Feeling safe and confident to discuss what feels good and pleasurable with your partner is important.	Open and honest communication within a relationship is vital. It allows people to express what they want sexually and can clear up any misunderstandings.
	Ultra-thin condoms allow for a skin-to-skin feeling.	Promotes pleasure as a key ingredient for people to practice safer sax and be protected.

Opportunities to include pleasure in your conversation with teenagers about sexuality:

- Teach about pleasure for all bodies, not just in the context of ejaculation and penile–vaginal intercourse.
- Normalise exploration, curiosity and pleasure. For example: "it can take time for you to find out what feels good."
- Discuss consent as a tool facilitating both safety and pleasure. For example: "when you know what your partner enjoys and they know what you like, you can have a much more satisfying experience."
- Establish the expectation in your communication that sex should feel good.
- Teach the anatomy of pleasure and not just the anatomy of reproduction. For example, include information about the clitoris or that different body parts can feel pleasurable when we are sexually aroused.
- Discuss pleasure as a common reason to have sex.
- Acknowledge that many people feel concerned about being uncomfortable using a condom and provide tips for increasing pleasure. For example, placing one or two drops of lube inside of the condom.
- Talk about masturbation (self-pleasure) as a healthy activity.
- Include non-penetrative sex acts in your definition of sex.

REFERENCE LIST

Barrett, M. (2019). Acknowledging pleasure in sexuality education. *The ETR Blog*. Retrieved May 29, 2021, from https://www.etr.org/blog/acknowledging-pleasure-in-sexuality-education/

University of Amsterdam. (2017). *Ellen Laan, professor of biopsychosocial determinants of sexual health*. University of Amsterdam. Retrieved May 29, 2021, from https://www.uva.nl/en/content/news/professor-appointments/2017/01/ellen-laan-professor-of-biopsychosocial-determinants-of-sexual-health.html?1576780769671&cb

Urban, R. (2018). Why pleasure should be part of sex education in schools. *Family Planning Victoria*. Retrieved May 29, 2021, from https://www.fpv.org.au/blog/why-pleasure-should-be-part-of-sex-ed

CHAPTER 12
Gender and sexual identity

Our understanding of gender and sexual identity, like many other aspects of sexuality, is continuously expanding. Although history and anthropological studies are filled with examples of diverse gender expressions, gender norms, sexual identities and diverse human sexual practices, the current status quo is based on a narrow idea of heteronormativity. Heteronormativity is the idea that sex and romantic relationships are only normal between a cis-gendered (refer to page x for definition) woman and a cis-gendered (refer to page x for definition) man, that sex involves a penis penetrating a vagina and that the other forms and expressions of sexuality and gender are not normal, or at least not as normal as this one!

The problem with heteronormativity is the narrow concept of 'normality' which is attached to it. Heterosexual people are as normal as homosexual people or people with other sexual identities. People have always expressed their gender and sexuality in many ways. As our understanding of human sexuality and gender matures, we are discovering even more ways that people can express themselves beyond the traditional descriptions. Facebook now has about 60 options for users' gender. Whether labels are useful or not is a discussion for another time (or book), but the point is that human sexuality is much more diverse than most people think.

Don't hold on to your idea of your child's sexual orientation or gender identity. We all make assumptions about other people, including our children. So, if the sex which was assigned at birth to your child is female, hold that idea loosely. As they grow up they may tell you their gender is different than the sex that was assigned to them at birth (biological makeup).

Here are some definitions about gender and sexual identity, as they can get confused (Monash University, n.d.).

SEX

Sex generally refers to the chromosomal and anatomical characteristics related with biological sex. A sex of the person is usually assigned at birth by medical professionals or parents based on the genitals of the baby.

GENDER

Gender is the socio-cultural aspect of being male, female or other genders and traditionally was assumed based on the sex of the person. Gender presentation is how a person expresses their gender using signs and signals such as clothing, physical appearance and even behaviour and mannerisms. Gender expression is something we learn from our environment and is expected of us based on our assumed gender. However, a person's gender *identity* is an internal psychological state. It is a felt experience. Simply put, only the person can say what gender they are.

SEXUAL ORIENTATION

Traditionally sexual orientation has been defined as the physical/sexual/romantic way we feel towards another person based on their gender. It is different from gender identity. Gender identity is who a person sees themselves as on the gender spectrum (such as female, male, non-binary, gender fluid, etc.). Sexual orientation is who you are attracted to (e.g. gay, lesbian, straight, pansexual).

However, as our understanding of human sexuality depends, defining our sexual orientation only based on what *gender* we are attracted to seems inadequate because the traditional models of sexuality (Schoofs & Van De Vijver, 2016):

- Generally have a binary view of gender (we now understand there are more than just two categories of gender).
- Don't include aspects of sexuality other than what gender we are attracted to.
- Don't allow for different types of attraction or different types of sex.

Sexual configuration theory (SCT) aims to combine various aspects of sexuality to help us better understand sexual orientation (Schudson et al., 2017). It recognises that gender and sexuality are closely connected. Defining sexual orientation solely based on whether we are attracted to someone of the same or different gender as our own can be difficult, as people's ideas of what is similar or different can vary. Consider the following questions (Ambrose, 2014):

- (If you are attracted to men): Am I attracted to men because I am attracted to people with a penis? People who act masculine? People who identify as men?
- What similarities or differences beyond gender are important to me in a potential partner (i.e. is gender the only factor I consider when it comes to sexual attraction to a partner)?

Other aspects of sexuality that could equally be important for us include the following, and many more (you may want to think which are relevant to you, and in what ways):

- Levels of sexual attraction (from none to high)
- Physical aspects of attraction that aren't related to gender (e.g. smile, eye colour, body shape and size)
- The number of partners we like to have (from none to many)
- The age or experience of people we're attracted to in relation to our own
- Whether our sexuality is linked to power and where we like to be in relation to that (e.g. dominant, submissive, both or neither)
- Roles we would like to play sexually (e.g. active or passive, initiating or receiving)
- The kinds of sensations, fantasies and experiences we enjoy sexually

For most people these are just as important as the gender of the people they are attracted to in defining their sexual orientation.

One of the challenges I have heard from clients and others in my life is keeping up with the growing number of letters in the LGBTQIA+ term. Most people would like to be inclusive and respectful of others and use the correct terminology when referring to them and talking about their gender or sexuality; however, they feel it is difficult to remember and understand the numerous changes to this term. I remember the time when the acronym for sexual and gender diversity only consisted of GL (gay and lesbian)! But our understanding of human sexuality just like any other aspect of human sciences is constantly growing and deepening. I believe one of the problems with extending the LGBTQIA+ term is that it does not allow for the complexity of human sexuality, and it implies that sexuality, gender and sexual orientation are specific to a minority group.

We all as humans have sexuality, and our sexuality is diverse and unique. For example, some people prefer erotic experiences by themselves, such as masturbation, whereas others really enjoy partnered sex. Some might prefer solo sex sometimes and partnered sex at other times in their lives. Some people are not sexually attracted to others at all, or they are drawn to them but do not experience sexual feelings. Some people might be emotionally and romantically attracted to other people, and others may not.

As you can see, the landscape of sexuality is diverse and rich (Ambrose, 2014).

SEXUAL ORIENTATION VERSUS SEXUAL BEHAVIOUR

The kinds of people, roles or experiences we're sexually attracted to can differ from our sexual behaviour. For example, you may identify as a heterosexual woman but feel that you could be attracted to and have sex with women in specific times or under specific circumstances. Or you may generally be more oriented towards polyamory and multi-partnered relationships, but at the moment you are in a relationship with one person. Our sexual behaviour is not the defining factor in our sexual orientation (identity).

For example, the number of young adults who are attracted to more than one gender is around 40%. However, the number of young adults who *identify* as bisexual, pansexual or queer is around 2%. But much more than just 2% of young people have sex with people of more than one gender regardless of their sexual identity (orientation) (Ambrose, 2014).

SEXUALITY IS FLUID

Our sexualities are also dynamic and fluid. All aspects of them can change over time, although some can remain relatively fixed. This is true about your child's sexuality as well. If they identify as pansexual (attracted to others regardless of their gender) because they feel that is more representative of who they are sexually, it is true for them at this point in time. They may identify with a different label in a few years, but that doesn't mean their sexuality in their early years was necessarily confused. Sometimes throughout time we find identity labels that feel more true and accurate, and sometimes due to the fluid and flexible nature of our sexuality we no longer identify with the previous label. It is important to note that some people choose to have no label for their sexuality, and that is a valid option as well.

Another important note is that we cannot consciously change our sexuality. It can organically change over time, but we can't cause it to change (Ambrose, 2014).

TALKING TO YOUR CHILD ABOUT SEXUAL ORIENTATION

There is no need to ask your child what their sexual orientation is, but rather explore their thoughts and feelings with them as they develop. Things will become clear when they do and as they get to know themselves better and experience the world. For your child discovering their sexual orientation may be a lifelong evolving process or a quick one. It is important that we provide a safe environment for them to be able to talk about their sexual orientation when they are ready.

So, rather than one serious, formal 'sit-down' conversation about gender identity and sexual orientation, look for small opportunities. When your kids are in the car, your daughter might tell you her friend is in a new relationship with someone. That can become an opportunity to ask questions such as "What is the name of Rachel's partner?" (instead of "What is the name of Rachel's new boyfriend?") or "Is there someone in your life?" (rather than "Do you have a boyfriend too?"). And to use the opportunity to talk about healthy relationships, you might say "What do you think about relationships? What age do you think is old enough to start a relationship?" and even "What does it mean for someone to be a good romantic partner or a not so good one?" The focus for that question is to provide the opportunity to talk about respect, trust, compassion, empathy, etc. and to include inclusive language rather than making assumptions (Stancil, 2019).

Then, as your conversations progress, you can gauge where your child is with their own feelings, what level they are at in understanding and offer that reassurance to them that you are open to listening. I also think it is important to thank your kids for sharing their thoughts with you. Remember, your kids do not have to share this stuff with you. If they learn it's not safe, they will seek out other avenues to get information.

Unfortunately, due to discrimination and ignorant behaviours of many people, children who are gender or sexually diverse (non-cisgendered, non-heterosexual) are five times more at risk of attempting suicide (National LGBTI Health Alliance, 2020). Providing a safe space for your child to talk about their gender and sexual identity can literally save their lives.

What is not said is sometimes as important as what is said. For example, maybe on TV two men kiss and Uncle Joe makes a rude joke. If you never refer back to that, your child might hear the message that your family is not accepting of people who are gay or lesbian. So, maybe following up with your child later asking them about how Uncle Joe reacted (something like, "What did you think about Uncle Joe's words when he was watching TV?") Starting a conversation about it can create an open space for discussion. You can follow up with, "Can I tell you what I think about it?" You can take that opportunity to share your values and beliefs even in a simple statement like, "I believe people should feel free to find the partner they love and trust regardless of their gender." You could then talk about what love is, how it feels or looks and how to handle physical intimacy (such as kissing, touching, sex) when you are interested in someone. Again, this offers another opportunity for you to share your own values and beliefs and create a safe and inclusive space for your child.

Making sure you follow up with your child and sharing that they have a safe space to talk about how they feel is important. We often assume our children know we love them no matter what, but that may not always be the case. It's good practice to tell them you love them for the whole of who they are and tell them they can talk with you. If you are uncomfortable or a topic is triggering for you, it's a good idea to pick out a trusted adult you can point them to.

GENDER ROLES AND GENDER EXPECTATIONS

Read the following story (Vernacchio, 2014):

Alex's parents were going out of town for the weekend and Alex thought that would provide a great opportunity to have a little party for a few friends at the family's beach house. Alex called Chris, M.J. and Sam and invited them to the party. Chris asked if there would be alcohol at the party. Alex's parents did not drink and had no liquor in the house, but Alex said there would definitely be alcohol at the party. Alex went to the liquor store, but being underage and having no ID, there was no way Alex could buy the alcohol. A stranger, Pat, agreed to buy the alcohol for Alex and charged a $20.00 'service fee'. Alex gladly paid the money and Pat provided the alcohol.

Later that night, Alex, M.J., Chris and Sam were having a good time. Chris had always thought M.J. was hot and decided tonight would be a perfect opportunity to make a move. Chris never let M.J.'s cup go empty. After an hour or so of drinking, Chris suggested they go upstairs. Sam noticed that M.J. looked awfully drunk and that Chris was paying a lot of attention to M.J. Sam followed the pair upstairs and found M.J. passed out on the bed. Chris seemed scared and didn't know what to do. Sam told Alex, who made a call to Dr. Green to ask for advice. Dr. Green called 911 and Alex's parents. M.J. was taken to the hospital and was released a few hours later, luckily perfectly fine.

- What gender did you imagine the characters to have (Alex, M.J., Chris, Sam, Pat, Dr. Green)?
- What do you think were the factors which influenced your thinking?

There are no right or wrong answers to the previous questions. Although there are no biological gender markers for the characters in this story, when I do this exercise in workshops most people imagine Chris and M.J. as a heterosexual couple, with Chris being male and M.J. being female. The reason they give is Chris persues M.J.; that it sounds like a common scenario: boy/man gets the girl/woman drunk to pave the way to sex.

This exercise helps bring stereotypical gender scripts to our awareness. We all, naturally, make assumptions about people's behaviours, motives and traits based on a gender label they have received (or we assign to them). The reason I say naturally is that as humans we all have a natural human tendency to sort people into groups based on characteristics such as age, gender, race, ethnicity, sexual orientation, disability, etc. These unconscious responses allow our brain to process vast amounts of information about one another at lightning speed. We process approximately 200,000 times more information each second unconsciously than consciously. Having to process everything about each person we meet would be both overwhelming and likely incapacitating. Categorising it has a function (Macrae & Bodenhausen, 2000).

However, the downside of it is that we then pay attention to facts that confirm our assumptions and ignore or screen out facts that contradict them. How does this relate to gender scripts? Gender scripts are socially and culturally constructed concepts and codes of behaviour for a man and a woman in a given society (traditional binary understanding of gender) (Vernacchio, 2014). For example, in most cultures men are considered hypersexual and are expected to get sexually aroused regardless of the context, their mental and emotional well-being or the quality of the relationship. Men are viewed as 'hunters' and are expected to pursue women (in a heterosexual relationship) and initiate sex. Women, on the other hand, are viewed as intrinsically having a lower libido and are expected to respond to a man's desire (either accept or deny). Men and women who don't fall within this rigid view of sexuality are viewed as 'weak', 'broken' (men), 'sluts' or 'aggressive' (women).

Gender scripts influence many things from the way we dress to how we walk, talk, what kind of jobs we apply for, whom we socialise with, the way we regulate our emotions and whether we seek help when we feel vulnerable to daily chores. But what is wrong with this, you may ask?

Narrow views of gender and strict gender scripts can lead to increased risk of mental health, sexual dysfunctions and a greater sense of unfulfilment in life. Social pressures can often make us feel like we must conform to gender norms, which can prevent us from exploring things that would make us feel authentic or fulfilled.

Boys face significant social consequences, including social judgement and ostracism, if they deviate even slightly from the culturally accepted norms of masculinity (Fine, 2010). There's something *wrong* with a boy who likes pink. There's something *off* about a boy who doesn't like sports. Boys who go against gender scripts risk being humiliated by peers or shamed as broken by their adults in their life. Liking a particular activity or colour is not inherently associated with our biological sex and gender. These are all meanings we associate with them. For example, it is interesting to know up until the late 1800s pink was considered a masculine colour in many Western cultures (*Ladies' Home Journal*, 1889, p. 3; *The Journal of Education*, 1889, p. 187; Spofford, 1891, p. 265).

On the other hand, women's sexuality is policed in other ways. If the primary shame for men is weakness, for women it is often their sexuality. Women's sexual interest is viewed as something to be repressed. Women are expected to walk the thin line between being sexually available but not sexually open and expressive.

The majority of the challenges my clients face in relation to their sexuality (erectile dysfunction, sexual pain, rapid ejaculation, relationship conflicts) are directly or indirectly related to the gender script they have been expected to conform to. When society enforces strict gender roles for both men and women, it can suppress our unique identities and prevent us from expressing ourselves authentically (Vernacchio, 2014).

When boys are called 'ladies' or 'pussies' as a way to make them work harder, their ideas of gender roles, masculinity and femininity are being shaped. When a girl is called a 'whore' because she is sexually active or is assertive in expressing what she wants or doesn't want sexually, her view of sexuality, her rights as a woman and her future behaviour is being shaped.

DO WOMEN INTRINSICALLY HAVE LOWER SEX DRIVE?

One of the main gender scripts about female sexuality is that they inherently have a lower sex drive. Let's check this assumption.

We have heard so many times throughout history that women have lower sex drives than men and yet, despite this repeated assurance that women don't particularly have high sexual desire, in cultures around the world people have gone to extraordinary efforts to control female libido: female genital mutilation, medieval witch burnings, chastity belts, suffocating corsets, continuous insults about 'insatiable' whores, slut shaming, pathologising medical diagnosis of nymphomania or hysteria and continuous insults on any woman who chooses to be generous with her sexuality. It all seems a little bit strange to keep supposedly low-key female libido under control (Ryan & Jethá, 2010).

So, the answer to whether women intrinsically have lower libido than men is no. If they do it is because of how we teach them about sexuality. How with our language and interactions we sustain this constructed idea of low libido.

As parents, having awareness of our own gender scripts and the way we police them is fundamental is supporting our children to develop healthy sexual and gender identities.

Some tips on helping children develop a healthy sense of gender identity (Hoffman, 2021):

1. Encourage personal expression when it comes to toys. Introduce your child to a range of toys, games and activities, including those that are traditionally thought to be for the 'opposite' gender, as well as gender neutral toys. Research shows children who play with more gender-neutral toys (in addition to having conversations about gender equality) grow up to be more balanced in their views of gender and in creating a more equal world.
2. Use play and imagination as a way to define positive values and qualities. When role playing—with toys or imaginary characters—get creative and create scenarios that introduce a full range of healthy emotions and respectful communication and relationships. You can help your child explore their toy/character's emotional state by asking questions such as "Is she sad?" and "How do you know?" By doing so, you can emphasise the importance of being able to express a wide range of emotions, including compassion, care and collaboration, which is vital for a child's emotional development.

3. Challenge harmful stereotypes when it comes to clothing and self-expression. One of the ways to encourage children to be their authentic selves and break free from unhelpful stereotypes is to allow them to experiment with clothing and self-expression.
4. Find books, TV shows and media that have good role models. To help your child develop the gender expression or roles that feel true to them, it is important to create a nurturing environment that supports the cultivation of their identity. Read books or choose TV shows and media which role model values, interests, jobs and expressions of healthy, balanced gender identities.
5. Speak up when you hear disrespectful comments. Culture is the sum of things we bypass. When raising a child, we are not the only ones in the picture. Other family members, friends and people who interact with our children also have a large influence on shaping their sense of gender identity. If grandparents, cousins or family friends say something that doesn't align with your values, be sure to speak up in that moment. If not possible to address it in the moment, be sure to talk about it with your child soon after to help actively counter that message. So next time you hear someone call men or boys 'ladies' voice your concern about what message this is sending your child and other children present.
6. Identify positive role models. Identify role models in the family, community, media or school who model positive, healthy respectful ways to express their gender identity. This could be a male relative who stays home to support a female partner at work or someone who has vulnerable, respectful, open conversations with their family and friends. Use these role models as opportunities to have conversations about healthy masculinity/femininity/gender expression.
7. Walk the walk. There is nothing more powerful than your actions. The best way to show your child how to grow up to be a respectful, healthy, authentic person is to role model those qualities. Be mindful of the comments you make or the jokes you tell. What type of gender roles and expressions do you personally display? Are they the ones you would like

your child to adopt? The key here is being intentional in the way we interact with our children and people around us and to have an awareness of the impact it can have.

Young people with a disability

Parents and kids with a disability may face added concerns when talking about sex. But according to the Sexuality Education Counselling and Consultancy Agency (SECCA) the questions and concerns of people with a disability have around sex is not different from others (WA Health, 2018).

In society, sex and disability remain one of the greatest taboos. Mainstream media often portrays disabled individuals as non-sexual beings, making it difficult for non-disabled individuals to understand that people with disabilities have sexual needs and desires and can maintain intimate relationships just like everyone else. However, people with disabilities have the same desires and needs as able-bodied individuals and are capable of forming deeply connected and fulfilling relationships, including sexual ones. It's important to recognise that young people, whether living with a disability or not, and regardless of their sexual orientation, have a natural desire to explore their sexuality. Exploring sexuality, intimacy and relationships is a basic human right, and young people with disabilities have the same right and need to do so. Unfortunately, they may face additional barriers and may find it difficult to express their wants and needs.

As parents and carers of a young person with a disability you may feel uncomfortable with the idea of your young person exploring their sexuality or having sex. You may want to protect them from getting hurt, as they may have some vulnerabilities due to their physical or cognitive disability. I invite you to re-evaluate your assumptions about sex and disability. You can do this with the support of a qualified therapist or on your own. Although you may be very supportive of your child, you may be influenced by overt and covert messages from society about sexuality and who can and cannot have sex or be viewed as sexual/sexy/desirable.

It can be hard for young people to find the courage to ask about sex and sexuality. They may not know how to begin. Young people with a disability have often had limited access to inclusive sex education, which makes it harder for them to talk about sexuality. They might also feel ashamed or embarrassed. They may lack confidence or have low self-esteem.

Due to societal messages that people with a disability are non-sexual or not desirable young people with a disability tend to feel unattractive. They may have had a lifetime of illness, operations and interventions. As parents and carers, you can help them feel valued as a whole person by implementing all the strategies discussed in this book. If your child is old enough you can openly talk about the unhelpful messages society sends about disability, sex and intimacy. You can find role-models or resources that portray people with a disability who have fulfilling lives.

If you are unsure about the complexities of your child's condition and sex, talk to a qualified sexologist or trained professional in the area of sexuality and disability. In Australia there are multiple organisations and programmes parents and young people with a disability can access to learn more about sexuality in the context of a disability. I have included some resources at the end of the book.

REFERENCE LIST

Ambrose, J. (2014). The sexual configuration theory: Towards a cognitive neuroscience of human sexuality. *Archives of Sexual Behavior*, *43*(8), 1427–1450. https://doi.org/10.1007/s10508-014-0345-y

Fine, C. (2010). *Delusions of gender: How our minds, society, and neurosexism create difference*. WW Norton & Company.

Hoffman, Z. (2021, January 21). 10 Tips for raising children with healthy gender identity. *Healthline*. https://www.healthline.com/health/parenting/gender-identity-tips-for-parents

The Journal of education. (1889). Oxford University Press, 187.

Ladies' Home Journal. (1889). LHJ Publishing, Incorporated, 3.

Macrae, C. N., & Bodenhausen, G. V. (2000). Social cognition: Thinking categorically about others. *Annual Review of Psychology, 51*, 93–120. https://doi.org/10.1146/annurev.psych.51.1.93

Monash University. (n.d.). Understanding sex, gender and sexuality. Retrieved August 2023, from https://www.monash.edu/students/support/lgbtiqa/learning-about/understanding-gender

National LGBTI Health Alliance. (2020). Snapshot of mental health and suicide prevention statistics for LGBTI people [PDF]. *National LGBTI Health Alliance*. Retrieved May 29, 2021, from https://d3n8a8pro7vhmx.cloudfront.net/lgbtihealth/pages/549/attachments/original/1595492235/2020-Snapshot_mental_health_%281%29.pdf?1595492235

Ryan, C., & Jethá, C. (2010). *Sex at dawn: The prehistoric origins of modern sexuality*. Harper.

Schoofs, D., & Van De Vijver, L. (2016). An exploration of the impact of the menstrual cycle on cognition and mood in premenopausal women. *Archives of Women's Mental Health, 19*(1), 151–157. https://doi.org/10.1007/s00737-015-0538-7

Schudson, Z. C., Dibble, E. R., & van Anders, S. M. (2017). Gender/sex and sexual diversity via sexual configurations theory: Insights from a qualitative study with gender and sexual minorities. *Psychology of Sexual Orientation and Gender Diversity, 4*(4), 422–437. https://doi.org/10.1037/sgd0000246

Spofford, H. E. P. (1891). *House and hearth*. Dodd Mead, 265.

Stancil, S. (2019). Tips for talking to your kids about sexual orientation. *Children's Mercy (Kansas City)*. Retrieved May 29, 2021, from https://www.childrensmercy.org/parent-ish/2019/06/tips-for-talking-to-your-kids-about-sexual-orientation/

Vernacchio, A. (2014). *For goodness sex: Changing the way we talk to teens about sexuality, values, and health*. HarperCollins.

WA Health. (2018). *Talk soon. Talk often: A guide for parents talking to their kids about sex [PDF]* (2nd ed.). Department of Health. Retrieved May 29, 2021, from https://healthywa.wa.gov.au/-/media/HWA/Documents/Healthy-living/Sexual-health/talk-soon-talk-often.pdf

CHAPTER 13
Body image

You may already have experienced this yourself that a challenging and unhealthy relationship with your body can have a huge impact on your sex life. In order to connect with someone else's body, we need to connect with our own first and that is a topic we rarely receive education on as we are growing up. It is not just about self-pleasure (sexual and non-sexual) and exploring your own body but fostering a sense of love and gratitude for your body.

I have seen countless clients who stay in unfulfilling relationships because they don't believe they deserve any better: they are not thin enough or pretty enough or muscled enough to find a better partner. Or people who worry about how their body looks like when they have sex and therefore find it difficult (and sometimes impossible) to focus on their pleasure and the enjoyment of their partner, people who have sex only in the dark because they are afraid of their partner seeing them and who even believe they don't deserve pleasure because of their appearance.

There is a pandemic of body dysmorphia, or at least dissatisfaction with one's body, all around the world. The economy of many Western countries is based on selling products to improve our appearance, and the messages usually revolve around the idea that your body is not good enough and therefore needs to be improved. Young people and children are especially susceptible to such ideas.

Research suggests that preschool—and elementary-age—children are more dissatisfied with their bodies now than ever before, that girls as young as three already perceive heaviness as "bad" and thinness as "good," and that more than one-third of five-year-old girls restrict their eating to stay thin (Tatangelo et al., 2016). Nearly one in three high school girls, and nearly one in six high school boys have serious disordered eating patterns that require medical assistance (Stern, 2019).

As our child's parent, we have a unique power to shape their values in relation to self-image. While we are not the sole influencers on how they ultimately view their body, fostering an environment of acceptance and body positivity can help with the process.

Here are some tips on fostering positive self-image (Sunshine Coast Psychology, n.d.):

- Avoid commenting on your child's appearance.

A 2016 meta-analysis of 42 studies found that encouraging children and adolescents to lose weight or criticising their weight can lead to negative self-perceptions and disordered eating behaviours (Gillison et al., 2016)

Children learn to value those qualities in themselves which draw positive attention. A child who is frequently told how hard-working she is learns that it is important to be hard-working and will strive to be diligent. A little girl who is constantly told she is 'pretty' will learn to value that about herself.

Think about your values as a parent and what you want your child to value in themselves, then praise your child when he or she behaves consistently with that value. Remember that praising the behaviour rather than the child helps the child to develop a more stable sense of self-worth, rather than a self-esteem dependent on possessing a particular quality (such as beauty or cleverness). For example: "That was a generous thing you did" versus "You are very generous."

Talk to your child about how cool it is that her body can do cartwheels, that his fingers can play the piano and that their legs are so good at kicking a soccer ball.

- Model positive body image.

Avoid making comments about your own or others' bodies. No matter how you feel about your own body, don't body shame yourself in front of your kid. If you talk about your body in front of your kids, talk about what it can do or how it feels, not what it looks like.

Even continuous positive comments send the message that it is important to have a particular body shape. When describing yourself or others, focus on inner qualities or skills, rather than appearance. Similarly, take care of your body by maintaining a healthy life style.

- Model a healthy relationship with food.

The language we use to talk about food can have an impact on our relationship with food. Do not demonise certain foods as bad or too fattening. To encourage healthy eating habits, instead talk about whether certain foods are nourishing or will provide the nutrients that bodies need.

- Do not dismiss your child's concerns about their body.

Particularly as children reach puberty, they are likely to discover that there are things about their own bodies that they do not like. Listen to and validate these feelings. Reassure your kids that their appearance doesn't define them and that you love them no matter what size they are. Listen to their concerns about their appearance, body size and shape. Puberty can be a worrying time. For instance, if your teenager says, "I look fat in my clothes, no matter what I wear!" instead of denying or dismissing their feelings, you could acknowledge their feelings and say something like, "It sounds like you're feeling self-conscious about your appearance in your clothes." By doing this, you are validating their emotions and showing them that you are listening, which can create an open and safe environment for them to express themselves. You will be amazed at how a simple sentence like this can create connection and an openness in the other person to look at alternative points of view.

- Help your child to see themselves as a whole person.

We all have many different strengths, weaknesses, personal qualities and interests which make us the wonderful human beings we are. Talk to your child regularly about the inner qualities, such as skills and personality traits, that make them unique.

- Teach your child critical thinking skills to critique the media they consume.

Following certain social media accounts can reinforce ideas about beauty and attractiveness. Help your child make informed decisions about what media they consume (more on this on page xx)

LIST OF POSITIVE MESSAGES

Regardless of the age of your child there are positive messages you can communicate with them throughout their childhood/teenage years. Here are some examples:

- Your body belongs to you and you have autonomy over it.
- Teach them about okay touch and not okay touch.
- You have the right to say no.
- You can speak to me about anything.
- You have agency over your body and have the right to get upset if it is violated.
- Each body part has a name and a job to do.
- You have a right to privacy.
- Your body can be a source of joy and pleasure.

REFERENCE LIST

Gillison, F. B., Lorenc, A. B., Sleddens, E. F. C., Williams, S. L., & Atkinson, L. (2016). Can it be harmful for parents to talk to their child about their weight? A meta-analysis. *Preventive Medicine, 93*, 135–146. https://doi.org/10.1016/j.ypmed.2016.10.002

Stern, J. (2019, January 25). Child body image: How to help your kid develop a healthy relationship with their body. *Slate.* https://slate.com/human-interest/2019/01/child-body-image-advice-weight-shaming.html

Sunshine Coast Psychology. (n.d.). *Fostering positive body image in your children.* https://www.sunshine-coast-psychology.com.au/Blog/Articles-374/FosteringPositiveBodyImageinYourChildren-459/

Tatangelo, G., McCabe, M., Mellor, D., & Mealey, A. (2016). A systematic review of body dissatisfaction and sociocultural messages related to the body among preschool children. *Body Image, 18*, 86–95. https://doi.org/10.1016/j.bodyim.2016.06.003

CHAPTER 14
Age-based tips for conversations

Start talking about sexuality soon and often.

Do not wait for your children to ask questions.

Be an approachable parent, make yourself available, and listen without judgement.

Create safety in your interactions about non-sex-related topics.

BIRTH TO 2 YEARS

- Start using the right names for body parts: vulva, vagina, breasts, nipples, clitoris, penis, scrotum, testes. This will help you get used to using these words comfortably before they get older. As I mentioned before using the right words helps avoid confusion and gives children tools to communicate about their needs if something is going wrong.
- You can use bath time to name body parts as you wash your child. "Now I am washing your arm and your hand. Now I am washing your chest. Now I am washing your vulva."
- Pay attention to your kid's non-verbal communication. Do they want to be held/kissed? If you are playfully tickling your child and they start to show signs that they don't like it, stop. This is one way of teaching kids about consent and that they have autonomy over their body. Even babies as young as a few months communicate with us about what feels comfortable for them and what is unpleasant. Get curious about your child's non-verbal communication and respond accordingly.

2–5 YEARS

- Read age-appropriate books to your child about gender- and sexuality-related topics. (There is a list of age-appropriate books on page xx.)
- Teach kids every part of the body has a name and its own 'job' to do. You can point out that most people have body parts that are the same and some body parts that are different.
- Teach them about 'okay touch' and' not okay touch'. You can tell younger kids that an 'okay touch' is one that feels nice, that you want more of and a 'not okay touch' is one that makes you feel sad or scared or uncomfortable. I personally don't think teaching kids that there are some parts of the body that others can touch and some parts that are 'private' is very helpful when it comes to preventing sexual abuse. As we know sexual abuse starts with non-genital touch; however, in most cases children can tell/feel that something about the touch is not right.
- Teach your child that it is never okay for someone to touch them (anywhere) and ask them to keep it a secret.
- Refrain from asking children under five to keep any secrets from another adult/parent. For example, "It will be our little secret!" seems like a harmless thing to say to your toddler when you give them 15 minutes more screen time after Mummy told them no and is upstairs giving baby brother a bath. However, children at this age don't have the cognitive capacity to understand the nuances of 'good' versus 'bad' secrets. As parents and caregivers, we want to keep our children safe no matter their age, and we won't always be there to protect and guide our child in every situation that may arise. "Let's keep this our little secret" is what a predator relies on a child doing. So, by normalising NOT keeping a secret we are giving them valuable tools to seek support when they feel something is going wrong.
- Respect your child's autonomy and need for privacy.
- Children at this age touch their genitals for comfort. If they touch their genital in public places you can tell them: "I know it feels good but this is something to do at home. In your own bedroom."

Age-based tips for conversations

- When they ask: "where do I come from?" you could ask them: "what do you think?" When five-year-old Sami asked his mum this question, Sally responded with a full lecture about reproduction. When she was finished Sami looked at her blankly and said: "I don't understand what you are saying. Sarah (his sister) told me she came from Ashford hospital. I want to know if I came from Ashford hospital too." So, before responding, always check their understanding or what made them ask the question to have a better context to answer their questions.
- Usually telling a 3–4-year-old that the baby starts as a tiny egg inside a woman's body (inside a uterus) is enough.
- 4–5-year-olds can understand that a baby grows in a woman's uterus and that you need a sperm and an egg to make a baby.
- When talking about how babies are born, include information about assisted fertility, as this is a very common way of babies being made. You can say: "Babies are born in different ways: a man and a woman get physically close and sometimes the sperm meets the egg and the woman can become pregnant with a baby, sometimes couples go to see a doctor and with the help of a doctor an egg and a sperm are mixed together and are put inside a woman's body."

5–9 YEARS

- Use books and start the conversation about how babies are born. Don't wait for your child to ask.
- Respect your child's need for privacy.
- Make sure your child knows they can say no to touching that they don't want.
- By age eight start conversations about changing bodies.
- Use opportunities throughout the day (movies, music, conversations with friends) to talk about sexuality.
- Remember, sexuality is not just sex. Any time you are having a conversation about gender roles, gender expression, intimacy, love, relationships, etc. you are teaching aspects of sexuality and intimate relationships.

Topics to talk about with children

- Answer honestly. If you don't know the answer to a question, this is a great opportunity to teach your child about reliable sources.
- Encourage your child to talk about what they have learnt at school. This is usually a good conversation starter to talk about what they know/think/feel about the topic of sexuality.
- Buy age-appropriate books and materials about sexuality.

9–12 YEARS

- Talk with your child about when you went through puberty. Share with them stories about how you learnt about puberty, the myths you had heard from peers, your feelings, fears and insecurities. This can help your bonding with your child as well as normalise feelings of insecurity and awkwardness around puberty.
- Talk about crushes and romantic feelings towards others. Normalise the experience. Feel free to share your own stories about your first crushes and your emotions during that time.
- Ask what they value in a relationship. Listen without judgement and get curious about their perspective.
- Tell them sex can be an expression of love or sexuality.
- Normalise masturbation.
- Tell them not everyone has sexual feelings and that is okay and healthy.

TEENAGERS

- Talk about the positive and negative aspects of sex. As I mentioned before just talking about the risks associated with sex can increase teenager's risk-taking behaviour. They are filled with sexual hormones, they see it on the media and hear it from peers that sex can be pleasurable and therefore would not trust a narrow perspective of sex.
- When opportunity arises throughout the day (e.g. watching a movie, listening to a song) ask: "why do you think people have sex?" The reason for this question is that most often in sex education, reproduction is the only reason

named for having sex. However, humans have sex for hundreds of different reasons. Having a conversation about this can help your child become familiar with the nuances of human behaviour as well as provide an opportunity to talk about more complex motivations for having sex, such as power and control, and how to navigate them in a relationship.

Table of some reasons people have sex (Meston & Buss, 2007)

1. I was attracted to the person.
2. I wanted to experience the physical pleasure.
3. It feels good.
4. I wanted to show my affection to the person.
5. It's fun.
6. I wanted to express my love for the person.
7. I was sexually aroused and wanted the release.
8. I was 'horny'.
9. I realized I was in love.
10. I wanted to achieve an orgasm.
11. It was 'in the heat of the moment'.
12. I wanted to please my partner.
13. The person's physical appearance turned me on.
14. I desired emotional closeness (intimacy).
15. I wanted the pure pleasure.
16. It's exciting, adventurous.
17. I wanted to feel connected to the person.
18. It was a romantic setting.
19. The person really desired me.
20. The person made me feel sexy.
21. It seemed like the natural next step in my relationship.
22. I wanted the experience.
23. I wanted to become one with another person.
24. It just happened.
25. I wanted to increase the emotional bond by having sex.
26. I wanted to keep my partner satisfied.
27. The person was a good kisser.
28. The opportunity presented itself.
29. I wanted to intensify my relationship.
30. My hormones were out of control.

31. I wanted to try out new sexual techniques or positions.
32. I wanted to feel loved.
33. I wanted to celebrate a birthday or anniversary or special occasion.
34. I was curious about my sexual abilities.
35. I wanted to communicate at a 'deeper' level.
36. I wanted to improve my sexual skills.
37. I was curious about sex.
38. I wanted to say 'I've missed you'.
39. I got 'carried away'.
40. I hadn't had sex for a while.
41. I wanted to make up after a fight.
42. I was drunk.
43. I was turned on by the sexual conversation.
44. I wanted to keep my partner happy.
45. I was curious about what the person was like in bed.

SEXTING AND DIGITAL MEDIA

Most youth use digital media, including pornography, sexting and social media. Teaching media literacy can help young people make healthy decisions about their sexuality. Here are some messages you can communicate with your child:

- It's normal to be curious about sexuality and to explore and express your sexuality.
- It's important to set the same boundaries, communicate and treat other people the same way in the digital/cyber world as in the real world.
- What you do or see on the internet is public. Even if you are alone and it feels private it can be seen and saved by others.
- No sent media/content can be retrieved or deleted completely. What you do on the internet is permanent; even if you think you have deleted it or it seems to disappear, it's stored in the computer memory and a server.
- Even if you're embarrassed or think you'll get in trouble, talk to me or a trusted adult if you see or read something on the internet or social media that upsets you.
- Real-life people aren't like porn characters or social media celebrities.

MASTURBATION

- It is a healthy and developmentally typical behaviour.
- It is a safer form of sex that can be done individually or with a sexual partner/s with their consent.
- It's a common sexual activity that can be done by any gender at any age.
- When a person is familiar with their own body and sexual responses they are better able to communicate their wants and needs to a sexual partner and have better sexual experiences with partners.

PORNOGRAPHY

- In Australia the average age of children being exposed to porn is eight years of age.
- It is not a matter of if but when your child views porn.
- It is important to talk to teenagers about pornography.
- Porn per se is not 'dangerous'.
- Your child should know that it is illegal for people under the age of 18 to access porn (in most Western countries).
- In the absence of comprehensive sexuality education children turn to porn, and this can be harmful.
- The purpose and intention of porn is not education, therefore it is not a reflection of reality. Pornography is created to cause/enhance sexual excitement, not to educate. One metaphor I use to help young people understand the difference is that pornography is like watching a Hollywood movie. If you want to learn how to drive you won't watch *Fast & Furious*, right? Because the purpose of this movie is to create thrill and excitement. Similarly, pornography is intended for sexual excitement.
- Being exposed to certain body types and sexual activities can distort people's view of gender, body image and sexual expression and lead to depression, body dysmorphia, etc. However, one point I would like to highlight is that these ideals are common in all entertainment media—not just pornography. So be mindful of how your child consumes any type of media.
- Teach your child critical thinking skills to make sound decisions about what type of media to consume.

CONVERSATION STARTERS FOR SPEAKING WITH TEENAGERS

These are some examples of the questions you can ask your teenager when an opportunity presents itself throughout the day. Please remember *how* you ask the question and the environment you foster has a much more significant influence than *what* you ask/say.

How do you feel about. . . . ?

What did you think about. . . . ?

What does our family believe about. . . . ?

Does what you just saw online happen in real life?

Why do you think that topic was presented that way?

What will you do if someone sends you a text that upsets you?

REFERENCE LIST

Meston, C. M., & Buss, D. M. (2007). Why humans have sex. *Archives of Sexual Behavior*, 36(4), 477–507. https://doi.org/10.1007/s10508-007-9175-2

CHAPTER 15
Identifying and responding to sexual abuse in children

One of our jobs as parents is to protect our children from harm. Any parent's worst nightmare is to find out their child has been subjected to sexual assault. But the good news is there are many things we can do to minimise the risk of sexual abuse in children. I appreciate this is a dark and difficult topic and you may wish to skip this part and come back to it at a later time or with the support of a partner or friend. There won't be any details about child sexual abuse, but there are some general references and case studies to help demonstrate the points.

CHARACTERISTICS OF CHILD SEXUAL ABUSE

It is not always sex—it can also include a range of sexual behaviours that can be physical, verbal or emotional. It can include but is not limited to ("Kids Helpline," n.d.):

- Forcing a child to watch a sexual act.
- Having any type of sex with a child.
- Persistently intruding on a child's privacy.
- Speaking to a child in a sexually explicit way.
- Showing pornography or naked pictures or videos to a child.
- Taking pictures or videos of a child in sexual positions.
- Sending sexual content to a child online or through text.
- Kissing, holding or touching a child in a sexual way.

Stranger danger is a myth—Children are usually abused by someone known to them. Many parents worry that sexual assault can happen when they are on a family picnic and a perpetrator is prying for his next victim. However, in the majority of cases, perpetrators are known to the child and the family. How can you use this information? It is easy to start to mistrust everyone when you learn about this piece of information. However, there is no need to be suspicious and be consumed by worry every time you ask someone to take care of your child/children. What we can do is to be vigilant and if we identify any warning signs, to take them seriously. I have had parents telling me, "I had this gut feeling that there was something off about this person, but I never allowed myself to think he was capable of harming my child." The other important thing is to take your child seriously. If they disclose anything about feeling uncomfortable around a particular person, do take that into consideration and unpack it further with your child. Never push a child who avoids a certain person/place to do something against their will. Of course, it may not always be a case of sexual abuse, but it is something that needs to be addressed.

Sexual abuse is generally not an isolated one-off incident—Sexual abuse is most often a gradual process (called grooming) where the perpetrator starts off by getting close to the child by buying them their favourite toy/ food, sharing of small secrets and creating a relationship based on secrecy and manipulation. Therefore, fostering an environment at home where children can talk about what is bothering them is key to sexual abuse prevention. The abusive relationship then escalates to non-genital, however, intimate touches. Many children at this stage feel/ know that there is something wrong going on. I have had clients telling me they knew "something was off" but they didn't know how to tell their parents. This is the reason teaching about 'okay touch' and 'not okay touch' to young children is very important. Also teaching older children to pay attention to how they *feel* in interactions and relationships with others is crucial. Children who have the language and know they can reach out to their parents, get out of the abusive relationship at this stage. However, children who don't know how to communicate their concerns or are worried their parents would react in a negative way can be extremely vulnerable.

Grooming can be recognised by looking out for signs such as ("Kids Helpline," n.d.):

- Singling one child out and treating them as 'special'.
- Taking an over-interest in a child and buying them gifts regularly.
- Arranging special activities or spending extra time with them.
- Isolating a child from other adults or children.
- Encouraging a child to use alcohol and drugs.
- Insisting on physical affection even when the child doesn't want it.

Threats, tricks or bribes may be used to keep the child from telling anyone about it—Teaching younger children that 'we don't keep secrets from each other' can be a very helpful way of keeping them safe. For older children and teenagers, explain that secrets that make them feel uncomfortable are not okay and that you can always help in situations where someone asks them to keep a secret that makes them feel scared or uncomfortable.

The effects of child sexual abuse can last a lifetime—Although many people recover from traumatic events, childhood sexual trauma has a significantly pervasive impact on a person's general and sexual well-being. The good news is children who have a supportive family recover from the impact of such traumatic events much quicker and with support are able to live healthy and fulfilling lives. If your child has been subjected to sexual abuse, don't hesitate to seek help from a trauma specialist, both for the child as well as yourself and anyone in the family who has been impacted.

Signs of sexual abuse in children

Your child might not (be able to) verbally tell you they have been abused, but they may say or do things that provide some clues. Although none of these can be used individually to identify sexual abuse, but in context and when a few signs are present, they can provide enough information for you to take actions. If a child is displaying any of these signs and they haven't been sexually abused, it is important you seek help, as these signs can indicate some other significant challenges in the child's life which can be addressed by support from a health professional.

- Unexplained accumulation of money or gifts
- Disordered eating
- Aggression, destroying property, substance use
- Excessive compliance or a desire to be overly obedient
- Poor self-image, poor self-care, lack of confidence
- Persistent sexual themes in drawing, stories and play
- Regressive behaviours (soiling or urinating in clothing)
- Running away, recklessness, suicide attempts or self-harm
- Sexual behaviour or knowledge that is developmentally not typical (refer to the traffic light model on page xx)
- Sleep disturbance, fear of bedtime, nightmares, bed wetting
- Not wanting to be left alone with a particular individual/s
- Changes in behaviour—withdrawn, anxious, aggressive or fearful
- Unusual or repetitive soothing behaviours (handwashing, pacing)
- Difficulty concentrating, memory loss or decline in school performance

Responding to sexual abuse
Just like physical and bodily emergencies, sexual emergencies are diverse and your response to the child affected depends on the context, the severity of the abuse, the child's age, emotional needs, whether there is imminent danger, etc. However, here is a list of sexual first aid that you can use as a guideline if a child ever discloses sexual abuse to you (Australian Institute of Family Studies, n.d.; American Academy of Child & Adolescent Psychiatry, n.d.):

- If a child hints even in a vague way that sexual abuse has occurred, encourage them to talk freely. Don't make judgemental comments. "Thank you for trusting me and telling me about this."

- Give the child or young person your full attention.
- Maintain a calm appearance.
- Don't be afraid of saying the 'wrong' thing.
- Accept the child or young person will disclose only what is comfortable and recognise the courage/strength of the child for talking about something that is difficult.
- Let the child or young person take his or her time.
- Let the child or young person use his or her own words.
- Show that you understand and take seriously what they are saying. Child psychologists have found that children who are listened to and understood share more and have fewer emotional problems than children who are dismissed or not believed. Responding without judgement to a child who is disclosing sexual abuse is very important to their healing from the trauma of sexual abuse. "I believe what you are telling me."
- Assure the child that they did the right thing in telling you. A child who is close to the perpetrator may feel guilty about revealing the secret. The child may feel frightened if the perpetrator has threatened to harm them or other family members as punishment for telling the secret. "You did the right thing to tell me. Thank you for that."
- Don't promise that you will keep it a secret. You may need to make a mandatory notification or contact the police or other authorities to ensure the child's safety. If they are not your child, you may need to tell their parents (if they are not the perpetrator/s).
- Don't promise that "everything is going to be okay." Unfortunately, as much as we would like that, things can get messy and out of our control. Not being able to keep that promise can damage the trust in your relationship with the child. If this is your child, you can tell them "I will be with you all the way and will protect you and make sure you are safe."
- Tell the child that they are not to blame for the sexual abuse. Some children in attempting to make sense out of the abuse will believe that somehow they caused it or may even view it as a form of punishment for imagined or real wrongdoings.
- Offer the child protection.

- Report any suspicion of child abuse to Child Abuse Report Line (in Australia).
- Depending on the type of abuse, you may need to take the child to a paediatrician, family doctor or the Emergency Department for a health assessment.
- Tell the child or young person what you plan to do next.
- Arrange to see a psychologist or a mental health practitioner who specialises in child trauma.
- Hearing that a child or young person has been abused is distressing, and this will be felt even more acutely if you are a parent or relative. It is possible that the perpetrator is known to you and may even be a family member. Services that are available for children can also help support family members and friends of victims and guide you through the next steps.

Traffic light model

This innovative framework is based on the original 'Traffic Light Framework' developed by Family Planning Queensland in Australia. I have modified it based on my professional experience (Department of Child Safety, Youth and Women, n.d.).

This framework uses a traffic light tool to categorise the sexual behaviours of children and young people to help:

- make decisions about safeguarding children and young people
- assess and respond appropriately to sexual behaviour in children and young people
- understand developmentally typical sexual behaviours and distinguish them from concerning behaviours

Although this resource is based on current knowledge and research, has been designed by professionals and I have personally found it very helpful in my professional practice, it should be used within the context of your own life, rules and regulations where you live and in conjunction with other relevant assessment tools. It is not intended to be used as a prescriptive tool to identify sexual abuse or 'unhealthy' sexual behaviours and neither does it cover all possible behaviours.

However, many parents and professionals have found this framework to help them make more informed decisions about the well-being of their children.

USING THE FRAMEWORK

The traffic light model lists examples of green, yellow and red behaviours within four different age groups. These examples must be considered in context. Many parents say they experience a 'gut feeling' when their children are at risk of harm or of harming others. This framework is designed to support that instinct by helping you make effective assessments and decisions.

The age categories deliberately overlap to demonstrate the fluidity and variable nature of development. The 13–17 age category may also be a useful guide for vulnerable young people, or young people with physical or learning disabilities, up to age 25.

All green, yellow and red behaviours require some form of attention and response, but the type of intervention will vary according to the behaviour.

Green behaviours highlight opportunities to provide positive feedback and information that supports healthy sexuality. Yellow and red behaviours require observation, education, increased monitoring or therapy. Sexual development is influenced by many factors. When using the traffic light tool to categorise behaviour, it is necessary to consider the current social, cultural, legal, community and familial context.

If you identify a green behaviour
Green behaviours reflect safe and developmentally typical sexual behaviours. They are:

- displayed between children or young people of similar age or developmental ability
- reflective of natural curiosity, experimentation, consensual activities and positive choices

Expressing sexuality through sexual behaviour is natural, healthy and a part of growing up. Green behaviours provide an opportunity to:

- positively reinforce appropriate behaviour and to provide further information and support
- form healthy and positive sexual relationships and keep their 'traffic lights' green

If you identify a yellow behaviour
Yellow behaviours have the potential to be outside of safe and developmentally typical sexual behaviours. They may be:

- unusual for that particular child or young person
- of potential concern due to age or developmental differences
- of potential concern due to activity type, frequency, duration or the context in which they occur

Yellow behaviours signal the need to take notice and gather information to consider appropriate action.

- Recognising that behaviour may be concerning is the first step in a process.
- Yellow behaviours cannot be ignored, and it is important to think through the options available to you. Consider why the behaviours may be being displayed and continue to monitor behaviour.

If you identify a red behaviour
Red behaviours are outside of safe and developmentally typical sexual behaviours. They may be:

- excessive, secretive, compulsive, coercive, degrading or threatening
- involving significant age, developmental or power differences
- of concern due to the activity type, frequency, duration or the context in which they occur

Red behaviours indicate a need for *immediate* intervention and action, though it is important to consider actions carefully. When determining the appropriate action, identify the behaviour, consider the context and be guided by:

- the identified risks or needs of the young person
- the potential or real risks to others
- laws and regulations in the state/country you live in

What if the presenting behaviour is not in the developmentally typical behaviour list?

The list provides examples of the types of behaviours that would sit within each colour category. If the presenting behaviour is not given as an example you can use the following questions as a guideline to make a decision about the child's behaviour:

- Is the behaviour consensual for all children or young people involved?
- Is the behaviour reflective of natural curiosity or experimentation?
- Does the behaviour involve children or young people of a similar age or developmental ability?
- Is the behaviour unusual for that particular child or young person?
- Is the behaviour excessive, coercive, degrading or threatening?
- Is the behaviour occurring in a public or private space?
- Are other children or young people showing signs of alarm or distress as a result of the behaviour?

List of behaviours: ages 0–5

All green, yellow and red behaviours require some form of attention and response. It is the level of intervention that will vary.

Green behaviours

- holding or playing with own genitals
- attempting to touch or curiosity about other children's genitals

- attempting to touch or curiosity about breasts, bottoms or genitals of adults
- games, e.g. mummies and daddies, doctors and nurses
- enjoying nakedness
- interest in body parts and what they do
- curiosity about the differences between boys and girls

Yellow behaviours

- preoccupation with adult sexual behaviour
- pulling other children's pants down/skirts up/trousers down against their will
- talking about sex using adult slang
- preoccupation with touching the genitals of other people
- following others into toilets or changing rooms to look at them or touch them
- talking about sexual activities seen on TV/online

Red behaviours

- persistently touching the genitals of other children
- persistent attempts to touch the genitals of adults
- simulation of sexual activity in play
- sexual behaviour between young children involving penetration with objects
- forcing other children to engage in sexual play

List of behaviours: ages 5–9

Green behaviours

- feeling and touching own genitals
- curiosity about other children's genitals
- curiosity about sex and relationships, e.g. differences between boys and girls, how sex happens, where babies come from, same-sex relationships
- sense of privacy about bodies
- telling stories or asking questions using swear and slang words for parts of the body

Yellow behaviours

- questions about sexual activity which persist or are repeated frequently, despite an answer having been given
- sexual bullying face to face or through texts or online messaging
- engaging in mutual masturbation
- persistent sexual images and ideas in talk, play and art
- use of adult slang language to discuss sex

Red behaviours

- frequent masturbation in front of others
- sexual behaviour engaging significantly younger or less able children
- forcing other children to take part in sexual activities
- simulation of oral or penetrative sex
- sourcing pornographic material online

List of behaviours: ages 9–13

Green behaviours

- solitary masturbation
- use of sexual language, including swear and slang words
- having girl/boyfriends/partners who are of any gender
- interest in popular culture, e.g. fashion, music, media, online games, chatting online
- need for privacy
- consensual kissing, hugging, holding hands with peers

Yellow behaviours

- uncharacteristic and risk-related behaviour, e.g. sudden and/or provocative changes in dress, withdrawal from friends, mixing with new or older people, having more or less money than usual, going missing
- verbal, physical or cyber/virtual sexual bullying involving sexual aggression
- LGBTQI+ (lesbian, gay, bisexual, transgender, queer, intersex) targeted bullying

Topics to talk about with children

- exhibitionism, e.g. flashing or mooning
- giving out contact details to strangers
- viewing pornographic material
- worrying about being pregnant or having STIs

Red behaviours

- exposing genitals or masturbating in public
- distributing naked or sexually provocative images of self or others
- sexually explicit talk with younger children
- sexual harassment
- arranging to meet with an online acquaintance in secret
- genital injury to self or others
- forcing other children of same age, younger or less able to take part in sexual activities
- sexual activity, e.g. oral sex or intercourse
- presence of sexually transmitted infection (STI)
- evidence of pregnancy

List of behaviours: ages 13–17

Green behaviours

- solitary masturbation
- sexually explicit conversations with peers
- obscenities and jokes within the current cultural norm
- interest in erotica/pornography
- use of internet/e-media to chat online
- having sexual or non-sexual relationships
- sexual activity, including hugging, kissing, holding hands, consenting to oral and/or penetrative sex with others of the same or different gender who are of similar age and developmental ability
- choosing not to be sexually active

Yellow behaviours

- accessing exploitative or violent pornography
- uncharacteristic and risk-related behaviour, e.g. sudden and/or provocative changes in dress, withdrawal from

friends, mixing with new or older people, having more or less money than usual, going missing
- taking and sending naked or sexually provocative images of self or others
- single occurrence of peeping, exposing, mooning or obscene gestures
- giving out contact details to strangers online
- joining adult-only social networking sites and giving false personal information

Red behaviours

- exposing genitals or masturbating in public
- arranging a face-to-face meeting with an online contact alone
- preoccupation with sex which interferes with daily function
- sexual degradation/humiliation of self or others
- attempting/forcing others to expose genitals
- sexually aggressive/exploitative behaviour
- sexually explicit talk with younger children
- sexual harassment
- non-consensual sexual activity
- use of/acceptance of power and control in sexual relationships
- genital injury to self or others
- sexual contact with others where there is a big difference in age or ability
- sexual activity with someone in authority and in a position of trust
- involvement in sexual exploitation and/or trafficking
- sexual contact with animals
- receipt of gifts or money in exchange for sex

REFERENCE LIST

American Academy of Child & Adolescent Psychiatry. (n.d.). *Responding to child sexual abuse*. https://www.aacap.org/AACAP/Families_and_Youth/Facts_for_Families/FFF-Guide/Responding_To-Child-Sexual-Abuse-028.aspx

Australian Institute of Family Studies. (n.d.). *Responding to children and young people's disclosures of abuse: A practice guide.* https://aifs.gov.au/resources/practice-guides/responding-children-and-young-peoples-disclosures-abuse

Department of Child Safety, Youth and Women. (n.d.). *Child safety practice manual: Working with children who display sexually reactive behaviours—responding.* https://cspm.csyw.qld.gov.au/practice-kits/child-sexual-abuse/working-with-children-who-display-sexually-reactiv/responding/resources

Kids Helpline. (n.d.). *Understanding child sexual abuse.* https://kidshelpline.com.au/parents/issues/understanding-child-sexual-abuse

Appendix 1
Navigating adolescence: answers to real-life questions from teenagers

In a survey of 100 people between the ages of 12 and 19 I asked young people to share questions they had about sexuality. Here are some common ones and my responses to them.

1. WHAT IS SEX?

When you ask most people, they tell you sex means a penis going inside a vagina, but this is only one of many ways which people have sex. Sex is any activity that can bring sexual pleasure for the person/people involved. It could be touching each other's bodies in a way that is sexually pleasurable. It could be kissing one another's bodies or using different body parts (for example, fingers, tongue, arms, etc.) to touch the other person's body parts in a way that is sexually arousing. Sometimes people use objects such as adult sex toys to please themselves or their partner.

Some people only have penetrative sex, some people choose not to have penetrative sex, for some people this option is not available, some people choose to have multiple ways to have sex. None of these groups are 'healthier' or more 'normal' than others. Anyone can choose in what way they want to have sex.

Note for parents: You can explore this further by asking your teen: What are some ways you have heard of people having sex?

Appendix 1

2. DO ALL PEOPLE HAVE SEX? (DO I HAVE TO HAVE SEX?)

No—not all people have sex, and not all people want to experience it. There are lots of different reasons people choose not to have sex. Some people do not have any sexual feelings (desire), and that is okay. Not wanting to have sex (for a specific period of time or forever) is okay. The dominant culture in most places around the world values having sex and particular forms of sex. This makes people feel pressured to have sex. Listen to your body, it can most often tell you what you want.

It is important to note that having a disability is not a reason for people not having sex. Anyone can have sex, although they may have some restrictions in mobility, cognition, etc. Disabled people do and can have fulfilling sex.

3. WHY DO PEOPLE HAVE SEX?

You probably have heard that babies come from parents having sex. That is a man's penis going into a woman's vagina. There are lots of books available that explain how babies are made. What I would like to talk about here is that making babies is only one reason people have sex. There are lots and lots of other reasons, for example, for pleasure, to soothe oneself, to feel emotionally closer to one's partner, to sleep better, to be popular, to feel loved, to control others. Of course, like any other human behaviour the reason behind having sex can be helpful or harmful to ourselves or others. For example, if someone has sex with others because they want to be popular, then they may put themselves/ others at risk of getting hurt (physically, emotionally and psychologically).

Note for parents: You can explore this further by asking your teen: What are some other reasons that you think people have sex?

4. DOES SEX HURT?

No. Sex should never hurt. If it does, it's a sign something is not quite right. Some people experience pain when they have penetrative sex. This could be for several reasons, but if that is the case and the person would like to continue to have penetrative sex, then it is a good idea to consult a health professional. Sometimes it is because they haven't used enough lubricant (it is a product you can buy from pharmacies and some supermarkets) or their body is not relaxed enough to allow for intercourse and sometimes the reason is more complex, and they need to explore it with a health professional.

Remember sex is not just penis in vagina. Sex does not need to include any type of penetration. If you or your partner experience pain with sex, stop! If both people would like to continue to have sex, then change the activity. Explore different touch on different parts of the body (not just genitals), kissing, stroking, etc. Sex should be fun and pleasurable for everyone involved.

One of the main keys to prevent a painful experience is to relax. Spending some time preparing for sex, talking with your partner about what you find pleasurable, having lubricant available (if you are going to have any kind of penetrative sex) can help the experience to be much more pleasant.

Being intimate with someone and having sex is much more fun when you're both into it. If you are both feeling great, you're doing it right! Unfortunately, research shows girls in heterosexual relationships (one male and one female) don't expect to enjoy sex as much as boys do. This is why having conversations about what you (both) want and enjoy or don't like is important. A girl's pleasure is as important, meaningful and achievable as a boy's.

If anyone is feeling discomfort or pain, it is not part of sex. Stop and check in with each other.

Note for parents: You can explore this further by asking your teen: What have you heard about pain in sex? (Many

Appendix 1

people falsely believe sex is painful for women. Assure your child sex should not be painful and if it is, they can seek help.)

5. IS MASTURBATION HEALTHY?

Yes! Masturbation (it is also called solo sex or self-pleasuring) is when a person touches their own body to feel pleasure and/or express their sexuality. Like sex, masturbation can involve touching different body parts and not necessarily the genitals. In fact, touching different parts of your body when you have sexual feelings can increase feelings of sexual pleasure. It is healthy and okay to experiment with touching different body parts. You might be surprised to find out some people enjoy touching their toes or ears when they masturbate. There is no right or wrong as long as you enjoy it (and no one else is being harmed by it).

Masturbation is a good way to learn about your body. It can also help you find out what you may enjoy in partnered sex (if you ever decide to experience it).

Note for parents: You can explore this further by asking your teen: Do you think people who are in a relationship still masturbate? (Answer: Yes, and it is healthy and okay to continue to do so.)

6. WHEN IS THE RIGHT TIME TO HAVE SEX FOR THE FIRST TIME?

The time really depends on each person, but here are some questions to guide you in making your own decision when you think you may be ready to have sex. You can ask yourself:

> Have I spent some time exploring my own body to find out what is pleasurable for me?
>
> Do I know which spots in my body feel good and which spots feel unpleasant to touch?

Am I comfortable with the thought of being physically so close and intimate with someone?

Do I know how to protect myself from sexually transmitted infections and/or unplanned pregnancy?

Do I know where to go for help if I feel confused/uncomfortable/overwhelmed by the experience?

Do I feel comfortable to say no to my sexual partner if the touch/activity makes me uncomfortable?

Do I know how to say no when a touch/activity makes me uncomfortable?

Do I want to do it because I really want to (or is it because I feel pressured)?

Does the other person also really want to do it (or do they feel pressured by me?)

Do I trust my partner?

If you answer yes to all these questions, then it is an indication that you may be ready for your first sexual experience.

A word of warning: Even when we feel we may be ready to have sex, when we actually do have sex, we may feel different. This experience is completely normal. If this happens for you, talk to a trusted adult (your parent or other trusted adult) and be gentle with yourself. Like everything else in life, sex gets better by practice. As we grow older, we can get to know our own body better, we feel more confident to ask questions from our partners and experiment with different things and find out what it is that gives us pleasure. No one gets it right the first time (or the first dozen times) and that is okay.

7. I DON'T HAVE ANY SEXUAL FEELINGS. IS THERE SOMETHING WRONG WITH ME?

Absolutely not. About 1% of people don't experience any sexual feelings; that is 75 million people in the world! Some of them identify as asexual. Asexuality is a healthy sexual orientation just like being gay or straight. Someone who is asexual experiences little to no sexual attraction.

Trust your gut and allow yourself the time and gentleness for as long as you need. You have your whole life to figure out who you are and what you want. You can have no sexual feelings now but may experience sexual attraction in the future. You can choose to have or not to have sex for a million valid reasons.

If you think you might be asexual, you can ask yourself these questions (Advocates for Youth, 2019):

- Have I ever been sexually attracted to another person?
- Do you want to have sex?
- If you want to date or get married at some point, do you want sex to be a part of that relationship?
- If you've had sex before, was it something you liked? Would you want to do it again? How were your feelings about the experience different or similar to your friends or partners' experiences?

It's okay if you don't have answers for these questions yet, or if your feelings are still unclear. Discovering your sexuality/sexual orientation can take time, and sometimes what you call yourself or how you identify might change. It's normal for sexuality to change and develop.

Having no sexual feelings or attraction doesn't mean you can't be in loving and fulfilling relationship/s. Some people who don't experience sexual attraction feel romantically attracted to others (of the same or different gender). Many asexual people want—and have—romantic relationships. They might build these romantic relationships with other asexual people or with people who aren't asexual.

8. HOW CAN I SAY NO TO SEX OR A PARTICULAR TOUCH?

- You can always change your mind. Just because you have said yes to sex or to a particular touch doesn't

mean you have to go through with it. As we experience sex, we find what is pleasurable and what is not. Even if something was pleasurable in the past it may feel different this time.
- Say "no" or "please stop" or any other words you like to let the person know you don't want what is happening. You don't have to explain anything if you can't or don't want to. Saying no is enough to expect that the person stops.
- Let the other person know what you do want: e.g. kissing, different touch, watching a movie, going for a walk or whatever it is that you want.
- It is okay to say no to sex or different touches and activities. Everyone has the right to say no.

It is as important to respect the other person if they say no to sex or a touch.

Here are some ways people say no:

- I like you, but I am not enjoying this particular thing.
- I don't like this.
- This sucks.
- I want to stop.
- Can I stop us here?

If you feel hesitant to say no because you're scared about the consequences, or about angering the other person, this is a different thing and is a real problem. That is a clear sign that you cannot give real consent. The best thing you can do is to leave and talk to a trusted adult.

9. WHAT DO I (ACTUALLY) DO THE FIRST TIME?

There is no ONE way or right way to do sex. Of course, there are some legal and moral considerations. For example, the age of people who have sex or the places people can or cannot have sex in, and these depend on where you live. If your question is "am I doing it the way I am supposed to?" or "am I doing it like everyone else?" then I can tell you there is no one way or right way. Sex is about exploring what feels good for us and our partner/s. We can approach it with curiosity and compassion. If this is all too wordy and abstract, here is a list that may help you plan and feel more prepared for your first sexual experience:

- Am I ready to have sex? (Go to Q 6 for more detail.)
- Is my partner ready to have sex? Ask your sexual partner if they would like to have sex with you. It may feel awkward at first, but if we cannot even talk about it then we are definitely not ready to do it.
- The place and time. It is important that you have a private place and lots of time (at least an hour) without being interrupted so that you won't feel rushed and tense when you have sex.
- Talk with your partner about what sex means for them and tell them what you want. The word 'sex' is too broad and could mean anything. If you asked someone "would you like to have sex with me?" and they said yes, what you have in mind may be to get naked and touch and feel each other's body with fingers and tongue and what they may have in mind may be to have penetrative sex. If you don't talk about it then you both may feel disappointed or hurt.
- Communicate with your partner about what you want. Many times, what we want changes as we experience sex. For example, you may start with the thought of just touching each other's upper body and face and as you experience it you may want to touch the other person's genitals. This is absolutely normal and is a big part of sex. The important thing here is to communicate that with your partner. Something like: "I would really like to touch your penis now, is that ok?" A word of warning: verbal communication is not always enough. Sometimes the body language of the other person tells us something different. For example, they may verbally say yes but you can tell from their face, body or tone of voice that they feel uncomfortable with the suggestion. If this happens, always double check and give each other options: "It is ok if you don't want it. We can do something else or just continue like this."
- Most people feel uncomfortable to be naked in front of other people. Some people think they are not attractive

enough or thin enough or athletic enough. Although it is not helpful to have these thoughts, they are very common. Remember, if you feel uncomfortable about your body the chances are the other person does too. Be kind with yourself. Everyone deserves and can have an enjoyable sex life. You don't need to look a certain way.

- Have lots of lubricant and condoms handy. Although you may not plan to have penetrative sex, you may change your mind. Use condoms on your or your partner's penis and any sex toys you may share. You can use lube for touching each other's genitals or for any kind of penetration. It does make sex more enjoyable.
- Relax! This is one thing most people said they wish they knew when they first had sex. The more relaxed you are the more enjoyable sex can be.

10. IS WATCHING PORN BAD?

What is porn, you may ask? Pornography is printed (like books) or visual (photos or videos) material that shows human sexual activity to cause sexual excitement. Accessing pornography is illegal for people under the age of 18 in some countries. There are lots of debates about if pornography is good or bad. The answer is not that simple. It depends on the way the person uses that material. If pornography is used to learn about sex it can be harmful. Porn is for entertainment. It is not a reliable source of sex education.

There are a lot of things in pornography which are made up and are not real. For example, the size of the penis or the way people have sex. In most porn people have sex without talking with each other, they rarely ask for consent (permission) which is not realistic. Sex in real life is lot more chatty with moments of laughter and awkwardness. Most often in real life people verbally ask each other for consent: "do you feel like having sex?", "Shall we. . . ?"

What you see in porn is not what most people enjoy in real life. Let's be clear, even if someone enjoys watching a certain type of activity in porn it doesn't mean they want it in real

Appendix 1

life. If you role model what you see from porn, it is likely that it is not what your partner enjoys. The only way to be 'good' in sex is lots of communication with each other. It can be fun and sexually exciting to tell each other what you enjoy and what you don't like.

Research shows that kids as young as eight or nine years are getting exposed to porn. This is harmful for someone who hasn't even started puberty. Although for some kids and early teens it can be exciting to watch something that is for adults, it can be very harmful for their sexuality when they are adults and can make real sex less enjoyable.

If you have been exposed to porn or have intentionally watched it and are confused or scared or unsure about what you have seen, talk to your parents or a trusted adult.

11. IF I AM A GIRL AND SOMETIMES FIND MYSELF HAVING SEXUAL THOUGHTS ABOUT OTHER GIRLS, DOES IT MAKE ME GAY OR BISEXUAL?

You may already be familiar with these terms, but just so that we are all on the same page, here are some basic definitions. There are many many more words that people use to express their sexuality. These are only a few of them.

Sexual orientation—this means what gender we are attracted to. The following terms are some examples of sexual orientation.

Gay—a man who is attracted to men (this term is also used for women, so women who are attracted to other women).

Heterosexual—A woman who is attracted to men (this is also used for men: men who are attracted to women).

Bisexual: Men who are attracted to both men and women (same for women: women who are attracted to both men and women).

So, back to the question: does fantasising about girls, if you are a girl and mostly attracted to guys, make you gay or bi? The answer is you could be both or neither. I know, it is confusing. The thing is the world of sex and sexuality is much more complex (and interesting) than most people think. You could be gay, you could be bi or you could be heterosexual (also known as straight). Sexual orientation is fluid. It means your attraction to others may change over time. Another thing is that being attracted to a gender for a short period of time does not tell much about your sexual orientation. Especially in teenage years (and for some people in their adulthood) people experience different types of sex and relationships to find out what the right one is for them, so if you feel confused about your sexual orientation, don't freak out! It is a common experience.

12. AM I NORMAL?

Most people ask this question about their sexuality at some point in their life. I have worked with many clients who come to me to find out if their sexual attraction, fantasy or behaviour is normal. Before answering this question, I would like to invite you to think about some other questions: What does normal mean? Who defines normal? Is normal a good thing or a bad thing?

Spend a few minutes now and jot down your answers here (it will be interesting to come back to them in the future) or keep a mental note.

What does normal mean? The dictionary defines normal as "conforming to a standard. Something which is typical or expected" (Merriam-Webster, n.d.).

My experience of what people mean by asking if they are normal is: "Do most people have the same experience as me?" And when I dig a bit deeper what they really want to find out is: "If people found out about my attraction/behaviour/fantasy would they ridicule me, bully me or even worse, discriminate against me?"

Why is it important to answer these questions? Because most sexual attraction/behaviours and fantasies are more common than we think. So, in that sense all sexual attraction/behaviours and fantasies are 'normal'. But this does not mean that what a person is experiencing is healthy, functional or beneficial for them or the people involved. For example, compulsive masturbation (when a person feels they have to masturbate a large number of times during the day and they feel it is out of their control) is a common experience. However, this behaviour can be very harmful for the person and can have negative effects on their personal or professional life.

The question I encourage you to ask is: is this behaviour/attraction/fantasy healthy for me? Does it support my growth as a human? Does it harm anyone? Is it enjoyable for me and all the people involved? Does it make me fulfilled?

13. HOW DO I KNOW IF THE OTHER PERSON IS INTERESTED IN HAVING SEX WITH ME?

It may sound nerve-racking and intimidating to ask someone you like if they would like to have sex with you. What if they did not have sex in their mind and get shocked by me mentioning it? What if they laugh at me? What if it ruins everything between us? What if they run away as soon as they see me naked? What if they think I suggest this to everyone? What if, what if...."

The list goes on.

If it is any relief, most people experience having these thoughts the first time they want to ask someone to have sex with.

Unfortunately, there is no way around finding out if someone is interested but by asking and paying attention to the other person's body language. Is there a chance the person says no and rejects you? Yes, there is a risk of getting rejected in all relationships (including sexual relationships), but there are ways to manage that.

14. I FEEL HORNY ALL THE TIME. IS THERE SOMETHING WRONG WITH ME?

Feeling horny is a physical reaction which is called being sexually aroused. You don't have to be touched to feel horny. It can happen by thinking about someone you like or seeing a romantic or sex scene on TV or without any obvious reasons.

Feeling horny or sexually aroused is a very common experience in teenage years, and since it is the first time you are experiencing this feeling you notice it even more. But not everyone feels horny and that is also okay and healthy.

During puberty (around the time you become a teenager) your body produces a lot of hormones that are related to sex, and this can make your body feel a certain way and your brain to think about sex very often (or all the time). This is a common experience. There is nothing wrong with you.

There are some myths around which gender is hornier, and many people think boys/men are hornier than girls/women and other genders. But it is not true. Girls and other genders can be just as horny. This myth can make people feel pressured to feel a certain way or for others to be ashamed to admit that they experience sexual arousal. For example, some boys/men may feel embarrassed to admit (even to themselves) that they are not horny all the time, or some girls/women may feel shame that they do feel sexually aroused very often.

15. WHAT DO I DO IF I GET REJECTED?

Rejection is trying to do something you want and being turned down or not accepted. It can make you feel sad, angry, disappointed or insecure. All those feelings are okay, and it doesn't mean there is anything wrong with you. It also does not mean there is anything wrong with the person who rejected you/your request. Remember, rejection happens to everyone.

Sometimes being rejected by the person you like or love can be hurtful and difficult. But just because they did not like you/your request doesn't mean no one else will.

So, what to do with rejection? First, accept your feelings. If you find the feelings difficult to manage, talk to a trusted adult. It is also important to remember that these feelings are okay and they won't last forever. Give yourself credit for trying. Think about the good qualities you have. Do something to release the thoughts/feelings: dance it out, go for runs, listen to your favourite music, write in your journal, kick a boxing bag, go for swims and hang out with your friends.

16. HOW DO I ASK FOR PERMISSION TO HAVE SEX?

Consent is when everyone agrees or gives permission for something to happen. When we're talking about consenting to sex, it means that everyone involved is happy to participate. They don't feel pressured, forced or threatened and can change their mind at any time.

Consent is more than just getting a no or a yes. It is about having a conversation about what everyone wants. These conversations show your partner that you respect them and you will not do what they don't want. This is a continuous conversation before and during sex. You can talk about the things you would like to try when you are chilling out together, having a burger or going for a walk. It doesn't have to always be before or during sex. In fact, people who spend time talking about their sexual desires with their partners in different times have a more fulfilling and satisfying sex life. If someone says "okay, if you really want" or "I guess so", it usually means they are not feeling comfortable to say no. Always pay attention to the person's body language and their tone of voice. If you are not sure, double check and give the person permission to say no: "I want to make sure that you also want to try this. If you are not sure or comfortable, we can stop or do something else."

Appendix 1

Here is a great way to remember what consent should look like. Remember the word FRIES (Bustle, 2016):

Freely given—Doing something sexual with someone is a decision that should be made without pressure, force or manipulation (someone who is drunk or high cannot give free consent).

Reversible—Anyone can change their mind about what they want to do, at any time, even if you've done it before or are in the middle of having sex.

Informed—Everyone is clear about what they are consenting to.

Enthusiastic—If someone is not excited, or really into it, that's not consent.

Specific—We consent to specific activities. Consent is not yes or no to all the activities. For example, someone may say yes to kissing and no to being touched on the genitals.

Here are some examples of asking and giving/withdrawing consent:

Asking for consent (Rare, 2021):

- How do you like to be touched?
- What are you in the mood for?
- Would you like it if we...?
- Would you like a bit more pressure?
- I'd like to go down on you. Would you be up for that?
- Shall we take our clothes off?
- Are you in the mood for some hot kissing?
- I'd love to have sex with you right now. Would you like to have sex with me?

Giving consent:

- Mmm, that feels nice.
- That sounds great, but I've never done it before so let's go slow.

Appendix 1

- OH MY GOD! YES PLEASE. THAT SOUNDS SO HOT!
- Can we start by kissing and then seeing how we feel about the rest?
- Absolutely!
- YES!
- I'd like more of that.
- Can you touch me here?
- Can you move your hand faster?
- I love this!
- Let's keep doing this.
- Don't stop.
- Keep going.

Withdrawing consent (saying no):

- I don't feel like doing that right now.
- I'm not into that.
- No, I don't like the sound of that.
- Stop.
- This is uncomfortable. I don't like it.
- No.
- Not right now.
- Leave me alone.
- I'm not interested.
- I don't feel well.
- Not sure.

Checking in:

- Are you having fun?
- How are you feeling?
- Does this feel good?
- Do you want me to continue?
- You seem uncomfortable. Shall we stop?

17. WHAT IS SEXUAL ASSAULT?

Sexual assault is when a person is pressured or forced into sexual contact without giving permission. It can take many forms, such as touching someone's body without their permission, forced kissing or forced penetration of any kind. These are only a few examples.

As a person you make important decisions about what (if any at all) sexual activity is right for you. Agreeing to sexual activity with someone (saying yes or giving consent) means that you have freely decided to take part in that activity. If you are pressured emotionally or physically, if you go along because you do not feel you have a choice or because you don't know how to get out of the situation, you are not giving consent.

It is the same when you want to have sex with someone else. They need to let you know that they really want to do it. If you are unsure how to ask someone for permission, go to Q 16.

18. WHAT DO I DO IF I AM SEXUALLY ASSAULTED?

- Remember, it is never your fault! Sexual assault is a crime, and it is always the fault of the person who committed the crime.
- Talk to your parents or a trusted adult. If there are no trusted adults around you, contact the police.
- Talk to a counsellor—When someone hurts you, it can make you feel many different emotions, like guilt, self-doubt and worry that it was your fault. This is normal, and many people find it hard to handle these feelings. A counsellor can help you sort out these emotions and start to feel better. With the help of a counsellor and your own strength, you can get through this tough time and move on with your life.
- Be kind with yourself—do something soothing for yourself: listen to your favourite music, take a hot bath with candles, use some essential oil, paint, go for a run or whatever else is comforting for you.
- If you are experiencing emotions which are difficult, know that they will pass. Do see a professional such as a counsellor or a psychologist to support you through this.

- You are not alone. Unfortunately, many people experience sexual assault. There are many support groups available. Find your local support group online or ask your doctor or counsellor to help you find one.

19. WHAT IF MY PARTNER ASKS IF I AM OKAY WITH A TOUCH AND I DON'T KNOW WHAT I REALLY WANT?

Sometimes, we really don't know what we want and that is okay. Often we just need a bit of time to sit with the question and think about the answer. Remember that you never have to give an answer straight away. You can ask your partner to give you time to think about it.

In a romantic or intimate relationship, saying "I'm not sure if I'm into this" is an honest answer and a sign of maturity. You are allowed to take a few moments (or hours or days or however long you need) to think about what is right for you.

Remember, everyone is figuring out what they like and don't like and being unsure is part of being human.

You can use these questions as a guide to decide whether you would like to go with the suggested touch or activity:

- How does the thought of doing this make my body feel? (Does your body tense up with anxiety? Does your chest expand?)
- Am I worried? What about? Is there anything I can do about this worry? (e.g. if I am worried about getting an STI, can I make sure we use a condom or other type of protection?)
- Does this align with my values?
- Am I excited about trying this?
- Do I have someone I can talk to, or seek help from, if things don't go the way I want?

20. CAN I CHANGE MY MIND?

Absolutely! One hundred percent you can! At any time. You can take back your 'yes' whenever you feel like you don't want to continue anymore. It goes the same for your partner.

21. THE FIRST TIME I HAD SEX, IT WAS BECAUSE I WANTED TO GET IT OVER AND DONE WITH. IT DIDN'T FEEL GOOD. I NOW FEEL STRESSED THAT IF I FIND A BOYFRIEND, SEX MIGHT BE VERY IMPORTANT FOR HIM, AND I JUST DON'T FEEL READY. WHAT SHOULD I DO?

Sometimes we are dying to tick off new experiences. Other times we feel we have to catch up to what our friends are doing or we will be left alone. If you ever feel any type of pressure to have sex, it is a good idea to take a moment and think about if that is what you actually want. You can go to Q 6 to see if you are ready to have sex.

When you are in a relationship with someone (or you are just with someone you really like) but you don't feel ready to do sexual things, it can be hard not to feel pressured. It is okay to do less. There will be plenty of opportunities in the future to do more (when you both feel ready) and if the other person dumps you because you didn't want to do what they wanted, they are not a good choice of partner anyway. A good partner is someone who respects your choices and needs.

And because you say no to one particular touch or activity it doesn't mean you have to stop everything. You can do things that both of you enjoy and find pleasurable. Remember, sex should be enjoyable and fun.

22. I'VE HEARD SOME PEOPLE HAVE SEX WITH A FEW PEOPLE AT THE SAME TIME. IS THIS REAL? IS IT HEALTHY?

In order to answer this question, we need to understand a few words and terminology:

> Monogamy—Having a romantic and/or sexual relationship with only one person.
>
> Multi-partnered relationship—An umbrella term which refers to having a romantic and/or sexual relationship with multiple people who have consented to be in this romantic/sexual relationship. Some forms of multi-partnered relationships are open relationships, polyamory, swinging and many more.
>
> Group sex—A form of sex which involves more than one sexual partner.

So, the answer to the question is, yes, some people engage in group sex, which as I said before is a sexual behaviour; some people have polyamorous relationships, which may include having sex with two or more people at the same time, but not necessarily.

Is it healthy? Like any other sexual behaviour and relationship, the things which make polyamory, monogamy and group sex healthy are not the nature of them but consent, good communication, respect and awareness of emotional, psychological and physical needs of everyone involved.

23. WHAT IS SEXTING?

I would like to start off by explaining another word: cybersex.

Cybersex is any sexual activity between two people who are connected via the internet. For example, sending sexual messages to each other online or live video chatting where one or both people masturbate or are naked.

Sexting is a form of cybersex. Sexting means sending naked images or sexual text messages to another person in order to make them sexually aroused/excited. Sexting, like all other forms of sexual behaviour, has its benefits and risks.

Benefits:

- Some young people use sexting to build up their confidence to have physical sex.
- Cybersex/sexting allows partners who are physically separated to continue to feel sexually close.
- Some people use sexting with their partners to build up the excitement until they see each other to have sex.
- There is no risk of unintended pregnancy or STIs in cybersex, as the people involved are not physically close.

Risks:

- Once a message or a photo is sent out it is out of your control. There is a possibility that the content/photo is seen by others accidentally or intentionally.
- Unfortunately, sometimes people use the photos/messages to blackmail (pressure) the person to do things they do not want to do. For example: "You'd better do what I am telling you or I will send your photos to everyone."
- Sexting which involves people under the age of 18 (in many countries) is illegal and a crime.
- Sharing photos/messages without the permission of the person is illegal and is considered sexual harassment.
- If a photo/message is shared on social media or has been sent to others it is impossible to retrieve it completely.
- Sometimes people feel pressured to send nude images of themselves or are worried that their partner or crush might not talk to them if they do not do it. But this, like any other sexual activity, needs to be consensual. It means the two people really want to do it and are both aware of the risks.

It is important to know that sexting, like any other type of sexual activity, requires consent (permission) of all people involved.

Appendix 1

Deciding to send nudes or sexy text messages should be like deciding to have any other type of sex. Talk about it first. Don't send a 'surprise' photo of your genitals to anyone! It is disrespectful and against the law.

Once you have talked about it with your partner (or the person you want to send the photo to), be clear about what you are giving them permission to do. For example, you could say something like: "I don't want you to share this with anyone. It is just for you and please delete it once you have seen it."

Some things to consider about sexting (Stynes & Kang, 2021):

- Don't share pictures or videos of someone without asking for their permission first. Even if they sent it to you willingly.
- If it is a picture of someone under the age of 18 without their clothes on, it is illegal to have them and share them with others.
- Don't send pictures to someone you don't know.
- If someone threatens you about pictures or videos you have sent, talk to your parents or a trusted adult. Even if you have sent the pic/video you won't get in trouble for asking for help. Don't keep it to yourself. Threatening someone is a serious crime.
- There are laws in Australia to protect you from sexting. The law states that unless explicit consent has been given, sharing is a crime (that is, sending a 'surprise' picture to someone without talking to them first is a crime). It also applies to taking photos or videos of someone without their knowledge or threatening to share them. The laws become stricter if you are under 18 and even stricter if you are under 16 (to protect you from harm).
- If you have sent nude pictures of yourself to someone or you have received nude pictures of someone else and you are worried about it, talk to a parent or trusted adult.

24. HOW CAN I SAY NO TO MY FRIENDS WHEN THEY PRESSURE ME TO DO SOMETHING I DON'T WANT TO DO. I DON'T WANT TO LOSE THEM.

'Peer pressure' is what we feel when we think our friends, teammates, colleagues and so on want us to do something and we feel a kind of pressure to do it order to be liked by them. It is part of wanting to fit in and be accepted.

Anyone can feel peer pressure at any age. Adults do too, but it can be more intense during teenage years. You may feel a lot of anxiety to make sure you are liked and accepted by your friends.

If you feel pressured to do something that goes against your values, like laughing at a sexist joke, making fun of someone with a disability, or doing something you're not ready for, like drinking alcohol or having sex, it can help to ask yourself these questions (Stynes & Kang, 2021):

- Why do I want to fit in with this particular group?
- Why do I want to feel liked by this particular person?
- Is this (what they are asking me to do) what I want for myself?
- Will it make me happy?
- Could I get hurt or hurt someone else by doing this?
- Will I feel sick/weird/regretful about this?
- Will I be proud to tell my parents about this?
- Do I have a support person (a trusted adult) who I can talk to if things go wrong?

If, after thinking about these questions, you believe it is a good idea to proceed, then go ahead with it and discuss how it went with a trusted adult. On the other hand, if you think that the activity goes against your personal values and beliefs, it's okay to say no. It requires courage to assert yourself, but it is an act of bravery and maturity. If you're worried about your friends' reaction or any negative consequences, it's important to talk to a trusted adult as soon as possible.

Appendix 1

25. WHAT IS A CRUSH?

A crush is a special feeling you have for someone. People of any age can have crushes, but it is a more common experience for tweens and teenagers. It is different to liking someone as a friend.

It is usually an intense feeling you have for someone in a romantic way. Your heart beats faster when you hear their name or you are close to them. When you have a crush, you think they're perfect and fantasise about them.

Sometimes your crush is not aware of your feelings about them or it's not possible for you to be together. If you have a crush on someone, you may tell them or you may choose to keep it to yourself. Remember that it is possible that your feelings are not mutual, that the other person does not feel the same way about you, and that is okay. In fact, this is usually the case. If you feel rejected, remember that you are not alone. Check out Q 15 for tips on how to handle rejection.

Another important thing to remember is what consent (asking for permission) looks like in a situation like this. Stalking someone (following or watching them without their permission) is not okay—online, at school, anywhere. Making them feel uncomfortable is not cool. But writing their name over and over in your journal or fantasising about spending time with them can be really fun (Stynes & Kang, 2021)!

26. HOW DO I KISS LIKE ADULTS DO?

Kissing, like other types of intimate activities, is a unique and personal experience. Everyone kisses in their own way. You can get good at kissing by being thoughtful and considerate with your partner (Stynes & Kang, 2021). Ask them if they like less or more pressure, or where on their body they like to be kissed. Pay attention to their body language. Do they pull back when you kiss them or lean in even more? Do they return the kiss by kissing back or touching you back? Also, think about the ways you would like to be kissed and try to create that feeling for your partner, but be open to feedback.

27. HOW DO I KNOW IF THE OTHER PERSON IS OKAY WITH KISSING?

Romantic kissing can happen in different ways. Some people just fall into it naturally, while others ask first. It's a good idea to ask out loud so there's no confusion about what the other person wants. But there are other ways you can do it too, like leaning in and waiting to see if they lean in too. If they don't, it means they're not interested. If they do, it means they are.

If you're already kissing and suddenly feel unsure if the other person is okay, it's important to pause and ask them if they're okay with what's happening. This shows that you care about their feelings and want them to feel safe.

If you're touching the other person while you're kissing, pay attention to their body language and ask them if they're okay with it. It's important to remember that everyone, regardless of their gender, should ask for consent. Being considerate and kind is important for everyone.

REFERENCE LIST

Advocates for Youth. (2019). *In their own words: The importance of integrated services for youth who have experienced ACEs.* https://advocatesforyouth.org/wp-content/uploads/2019/03/ITIMB-ACE.pdf

Bustle. (2016). *Planned parenthood graphic uses fries to explain consent in a way anyone can understand.* www.bustle.com/articles/178198-planned-parenthood-graphic-uses-fries-to-explain-consent-in-a-way-anyone-can-understand

Merriam-Webster. (n.d.). Normal. *Merriam-Webster.com dictionary.* www.merriam-webster.com/dictionary/normal

Rare, R. (2021). *Sex ed: A belated guide for adults.* Bloomsbury.

Stynes, Y., & Kang, M. (2021). *Welcome to consent: How to say no, when to say yes and everything in between.* Hardie Grant Children's Publishing.

Appendix 2
List of age-appropriate sexuality books for children and young people

3–5-YEAR-OLDS

Everybody Thought I Was a Boy! by Anisa Varasteh and Sholeh Pardakhtim; 2018

What Makes a Baby by Corey Silverberg; 2012

The Amazing True Story of How Babies Are Made by Fiona Katauskas; 2015

Introducing Teddy: A Gentle Story About Gender and Friendship by Jessica Walton; 2016

And Tango Makes Three by Justin Richardson and Peter Parnell; 2005

King and King by Linda de Haan; 2000

No Means No by Jayneen Sanders; 2015

My Body! What I say Goes! by Jayneen Sanders; 2016

My Underpants Rule by Kate and Rod Power; 2014

Everyone's Got a Bottom Years by Tess Rowley and Family Planning Queensland; 2007

The Family Book by Todd Parr; 2010

5–10-YEAR-OLDS

It's So Amazing by Robie H. Harris; 1999

Hair in Funny Places by Babette Cole; 1999

Secret Girls' Business by Fay Angelo, Heather Pritchard and Rose Stewart; 2004

Secret Boys' Business by Fay Angelo, Heather Pritchard and Rose Stewart; 2011

And Tango Makes Three by Justin Richardson and Peter Parnell; 2005

King and King by Linda de Haan; 2000

Sex is a Funny Word by Corey Silverberg; 2015

Girl Stuff for Girls Aged 8–12 by Kaz Cooke; 2016

Growing Up Great!: The Ultimate Puberty Book for Boys by Scott Todnem; 2019

Girlwise—A Guide to Taking Care of Your Body by Sharon Witt; 2014

My Body! What I Say Goes! by Jayneen Sanders; 2016

My Underpants Rule by Kate and Rod Power; 2014

Everyone's Got a Bottom Years by Tess Rowley and Family Planning Queensland; 2007

Matilda Learns a Valuable Lesson by Holly-ann Martin; 2011

Not for Kids by Liz Walker; 2016

10–15-YEAR-OLDS

Puberty by Western Australian Department of Health (free online book)

Kit And Arlo Find A Way by Ingrid Laguna and Vanessa Hamilton; 2022

Hair in Funny Places by Babette Cole; 1999

Relationships, Sex and Other Stuff by Western Australian Department of Health (free online book)

Puberty Girl by Shushann Movsessian; 2004

Appendix 2

Wait, What? A Comic Book Guide to Relationships, Bodies, and Growing Up by Heather Corinna and Isabella Rotman with Luke Howard; 2019

Puberty Boy by Geoff Price; 2005

Puberty and Special Girls by Fay Angelo, Heather Pritchard and Rose Stewart; 2010

Special Girls' Business by Fay Angelo, Heather Pritchard and Rose Stewart; 2005

Teen Talk—Guy Talk by Sharon Witt; 2011

Where's MY Book?: A Guide for Transgender and Gender Non-Conforming Youth, Their Parents, and Everyone Else by Linda Gromko; 2015

Special Boys' Business by Fay Angelo, Heather Pritchard and Rose Stewart; 2007

Girl Stuff for Girls Aged 8–12 by Kaz Cooke; 2016

Growing Up Great!: The Ultimate Puberty Book for Boys by Scott Todnem; 2019

Girlwise—A Guide to Taking Care of Your Body by Sharon Witt; 2014

15–17-YEAR-OLDS

Consent: The New Rules of Sex Education by Jennifer Lang; 2018

S.E.X.: The All-You-Need-to-Know Sexuality Guide to Get You through Your Teens and Twenties by Heather Corinna; 2016

Wait, What? A Comic Book Guide to Relationships, Bodies, and Growing Up by Heather Corinna and Isabella Rotman with Luke Howard; 2019

Dating and Sex: A Guide for the 21st Century Teen Boy by Andrew M. Smiler; 2016

Dating Smarts: What Every Teen Needs to Know to Date, Relate or Wait by Amy Lang; 2014

The ABC's of LGBT+ by Ashley Mardell; 2016

In Case You're Curious: Questions about Sex from Young People with Answers from the Experts by Planned Parenthood, edited by Alison Macklin; 2019

The sex education website scarleteen.com

A mobile app called Real Talk

Resources for children with a disability

- SECCA is an Australia-based organisation which supports people with disabilities to learn about relationships, sexuality and sexual health. They have great educational resources for parents as well as children. Their resources are picture-based and written in easy English to ensure access and understanding. They use anatomically correct illustrations to remove the ambiguity that often confuses or adds shame to learning about sexuality: www.secca.org.au/resources
- The SECCA app is a free innovative resource to support access to relationships and sexuality education for people of all ages and abilities: app.secca.org.au
- The TASCC Supporting Youth with Disability is a Canada-based organisation which helps anyone who cares for or works with a child or youth with disabilities: www.tascc.ca/supporting-youth-with-disabilities
- *Sexuality and Relationship Education for Children and Adolescents with Autism Spectrum Disorders* by Davida Hartman; 2013
- *Boyfriends & Girlfriends: A Guide to Dating for People with Disabilities* by Terri Couwenhoven; 2015

Index

abstinence-based sexuality education 14, 166–167
abstinence-only programmes 14
active listening: LISTEN acronym 98–100; listening skills 88–93; tips for 100–101
adolescence see teenagers; teenagers, questions from age-based tips for conversations 191–198
Ainsworth, Mary 57
anger management 84–86
anxious attachment style 60, 62
asexuality 217–218
Attachment Effect, The (Lovenheim) 61
attachment styles 57–64
avoidant attachment style 60, 62
awkwardness see barriers to sexuality education

barriers to sexuality education: discomfort with conversations 42–43; identification of barriers 27–34; overcoming 40–43
birth to age 2 191
body image 186–190
body-oriented psychotherapy 40
body parts, names for 191
books, age-appropriate 192, 238–241
boundaries 126–127; childhood experiences, impact of 131; communication of 138–141; definitions of 128; healthy messages 136; identification of 128–129, 133, 137; and Inner Leader 137; LIMITS acronym 137–138; okay touch vs. not okay touch 192–193; setting healthy 137–138; testing functionality of 131
Bowlby, John 57
box breathing 80
breathwork 80

communication: of boundaries 138–141; and emotional intelligence 68; larger context of communication 153–154; non-verbal 191; place, choice of 151–153; value-based communication 125; see also conversations
communication skills 87–101; about feelings 95–96; active listening 88–93; hurt of offense, mending 95; intent-impact 93–94; mirroring 96–98
connection see attachment styles
consent 226–228; at different age levels 159–163; FRIES acronym 227; teaching the concept 154–160
conversations: age-based tips 191–199; asking questions 153–160; conversation starters 198–199; parent/kid

242

Index

conversations 16–18; *see also* communication
Cooper, Glen 63
critical thinking skills 101–106
crushes 236; *see also* rejection, handling
cybersex (sexting) 196, 232–234

de-shaming 51–52
digital media 196
disability, young people with 183–184; resources for 241
Disney movies 19–20
disorganised attachment style 60–61, 63
domestic violence 15–16

emotional intelligence 66–68; applications in parenting situations 77–78; case examples 82–87; common emotions and possible messages 76; communication skills 87–101; critical thinking skills 101–106; emotional literacy 72–74; emotions, list of 73–74; identification of emotions 71; parenting and self-awareness 69–72; parenting tips 80–82; self-management 74–77; self-regulation techniques 78–80; and sexuality 68–69
emotional literacy 72–74
empathy 69, 87–88; and mirroring 96

feeling confused with thinking 72
female sexuality 179–180; sex drive 180–181

gender: definitions of 171–172; gender identity 181–182, 222–223; gender-neutral language 6–7; gender roles/ expectations 177–180; gender scripts 178–179; societal expectations 2–3, 20–21
Good Inside (Kennedy) 45, 63
Gottman, John 70
group sex 232

Hakomi psychotherapy 40
Harley, Chris 15
Hazan, Cindy 59
heteronormativity 171; *see also* gender; LGBTQI+ young people
Hoffman, Kent 63
home/family environments 18

impact in communication 93–94
intent in communication 93–94
intimate partner violence 15–16
isopraxism (mirroring) 96–98

Jung, Carl 31

Kennedy, Becky 45, 63
kissing 236–237

language: gender-neutral 6–7; word choices for sex and body parts 149–150
LGBTQI+ young people 174, 222–223; importance of sexuality education 14
Lovenheim, Peter 61

masturbation 197, 216
Mayer, John D. 71
media messages 19–20
Miller, George A. 89–90
mindfulness 79
mirroring 96–98
monogamy 232

243

Index

motivating factors for talking with kids 24–25
multi-partnered relationships 232
mutual trust 49–51

nature, grounding in 80
"no-talk" rules 17

over-protection 50

parenting: emotional intelligence, practical application 77–78; emotional intelligence and self-awareness 69–72; gender identity development in children 181–182; parental roles in sexuality education 4; parents as positive role models 4–5; questions and answers 45–46, 142–146; for secure attachment 63–64
peer messages/peer pressure 165, 235
pleasure: attitudes concerning 35; pleasure-based approaches 168–170; and vulnerability 141
pornography 197, 221–222; children's exposure to 3; positive uses for 3
positive alternatives to shaming messages 168, 189
Powell, Bert 63
pregnancy rates for teens 15
psychotherapy 40
puberty 194–195

Raising a Secure Child (Hoffman et al.) 63
Ray, Rebecca 98–101, 137–138
rejection, handling 225–226
relationship violence 15–16
resilience 69

resources 238–241
risk-based vs. pleasure-based approaches 169–170
risk-taking 50
role-modelling: and communication 139–140; positive body image 188; relationship with food 188–189

safety guidelines 18
Salovey, Peter 71
school environments 19, 153
secret-keeping 192, 201
"secret language" 150–151
secure attachment style 59, 61–62; parenting for 63–64
self-awareness 69–72
self-care 7–8, 44–45
self-compassion 43–44
self-image 187; *see also* body image
self-knowledge: attitudes 33–35; influences on sexuality 28–30; internalised sexual beliefs 31
self-management 74–77
self-regulation techniques 78–80
sensorimotor psychotherapy 40
Setting Boundaries (Ray) 98–101, 137–138
sex: definitions of 172; reasons for sexual activity 194–195
sexting 196, 232–234
sexual abuse 199–211; impact of 201; response to 202–204; signs of 201–202; Traffic Light Framework 204–211
sexual assault 228–230; of children 16–17; *see also* relationship violence
sexual configuration theory (SCT) 173, 173–174
sexual harassment 28

244

Index

sexuality: definitions 23; fluidity of 175; misconceptions about 15–16
sexuality education: foundations 48–53; importance of 13–23
sexual orientation 172–174; contrasted with sexual behaviour 174–175; conversations concerning 175–177, 222–223
shame/shaming messages 51–53, 167
Shaver, Phillip 59
SIECUS 15
sitting with emotions 78–79
somatic experiencing 40
square breathing 80
stalking 236
STIs (sexually transmitted infections) 15
"Strange Situation" experiments 57–58
strength-based approach 109–112

teenagers 194–195; age-appropriate books 240–241; conversation starters 198; Traffic Light Framework 210–211
teenagers, questions from: consent 226–228; crushes 236; desire 225; gender/sexual identity 222–223; kissing 236–237; masturbation 216; multiple partners 232; pain during sex 215–216; peer pressure 235; pornography 221–222; rejection, handling 225–226; saying no 218–219; sex 213–214; sex for the first time 216–208, 219–221; sexting 232–234; sexual assault 228–230; sexual feelings, lack of 208–218; understanding desire and changing one's mind 230–231; understanding the other person 224; what is normal 223–224
thinking confused with feeling 72
traffic light model 204–211
triggers: identification of 37–38; planning for potential 40
trust 49–51

values: core values 113–114, 119–120; defining values 113, 114–122; identification of 41–42; value-based communication 124; value-based decision-making 113–125; value-based decision-making, questions for 122–124
vulnerability 140–141

Wiseman, Richard 97
women's sexuality see female sexuality

245

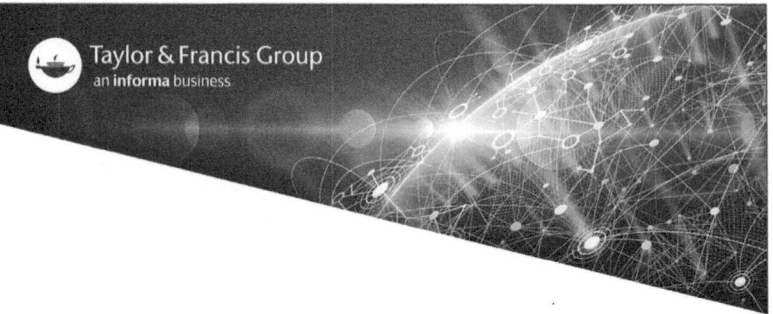